Jonathan A.J. Hyde
& Timothy R. Graham

Published by Family Doctor Publications Limited
in association with the British Medical Association

IMPORTANT NOTICE

This book is intended not as a substitute for personal medical advice but as a supplement to that advice for the patient who wishes to understand more about his or her condition.

Before taking any form of treatment YOU SHOULD ALWAYS CONSULT YOUR MEDICAL PRACTITIONER.

In particular (without limit) you should note that advances in medical science occur rapidly and some of the information contained in this booklet about drugs and treatment may very soon be out of date.

Updated 2001, 2003, 2005

Family Doctor Publications, PO Box 4664, Poole, Dorset BH15 1NN

Acknowledgements
Mairead Clune, Cardiac Liaison Sister, The Priory Hospital, Birmingham

Medical Editor: Dr Tony Smith
Cover Artist: Dave Eastbury
Medical Artist: Philip Wilson and Jane Fallows
Design: MPG Design, Blandford Forum, Dorset
Printing: Nuffield Press, Abingdon, Oxon, using acid-free paper

ISBN: 1 898205 79 5

Contents

Introduction	1
Your heart: the inside story	3
Ischaemic heart disease	11
Valvular heart disease	15
Diagnosis of heart disease	18
Non-surgical treatment	27
Heart surgery	33
Surgery for ischaemic heart disease	47
Surgery for valvular heart disease	58
Transplantation	64
Children and heart surgery	66
Surgery for rhythm disturbances	68
After your operation	70
Getting back to normal	75
Recent advances	83
Useful addresses	86
Index	90

Introduction

Although it is easy to say 'it won't happen to me', over 30,000 heart operations are performed every year in the UK. More than 99% of these fall into two categories:

- operations for blockages in the coronary arteries
- operations for disease of the valves.

What is not commonly known is that heart surgery has only been around for just over 40 years. In that time, progress has been enormous, both in technical and scientific fields, and in surgical expertise, all resulting in a better and safer operation for the patient. These days, most operations take less than three hours, and the total stay in hospital is about a week. There is an increasing trend for 'fast-tracking' patients through the system, enabling some to go home as early as three days after the operation. This compares with the 'all-day' operations and three-week or longer stays of not much more than ten years ago.

Most of us know somebody who has had a heart operation, but in the majority of cases you would never know to look at them, since the recovery is so complete. You would also be surprised at the large number of famous figures or celebrities who have undergone such procedures, since they carry out their usual roles as if nothing had ever happened. The whole point of heart surgery is to restore the quality of life to normal, not to restore a state of invalidity. It is usually possible to be back to a normal, active life within three months of surgery, and in some cases even sooner than that.

There is an enormous amount of fear and mystery surrounding heart surgery, most of which is unnecessary. This book aims to dispel some or all of that fear, and explain every aspect of what is involved, from how the heart works and suffers from disease, through the operation itself, and what to expect afterwards.

KEY POINTS

- ✓ Heart surgery is very common
- ✓ Most operations are routine and straightforward
- ✓ The aim is for you to return to a completely normal life

Your heart: the inside story

Every cell in the body needs oxygen and nutrition to survive, and these essentials are transported around the body in the bloodstream. The blood carries high concentrations of oxygen and 'food' to the cell, and carries the waste products of the cell's activity away from the cell. At the centre of the bloodstream is the heart, which acts as the pump and is responsible for the efficient flow of blood to and from the cells. In order to understand the disease processes that may affect the heart, it is useful to have a basic understanding of its anatomy, and how it actually functions.

How it is formed

The heart is a muscular organ acting as a pump that consists of four chambers: the left and right atria and the left and right ventricles.

Blood enters the heart through the veins into the atria, and is pumped out of the heart through the arteries from the ventricles. In fact, the heart is really two separate pumps that are independent of each other.

The left heart, consisting of its atrium and ventricle, carries bright red blood which is rich in oxygen and nutrition. This blood enters the left atrium, a thin-walled collecting chamber, through the pulmonary veins which come from the lungs. The blood passes through a valve from the atrium to the ventricle, a thick-walled muscular structure, which pumps it through the aorta to all parts of the body.

The right heart carries dark red blood which is low in oxygen and rich in waste products. The blood enters the right atrium (thin-walled) from the rest of the body via the vena cavae (superior and inferior), and passes into the muscular right ventricle, from where it is pumped back to the lungs via the pulmonary artery for disposal.

Thus, a closed circuit exists, consisting of the heart and the blood vessels, known as the circulatory system. This contains about five litres of blood, in the average-sized person, which is continuously recycled by the beating of the heart.

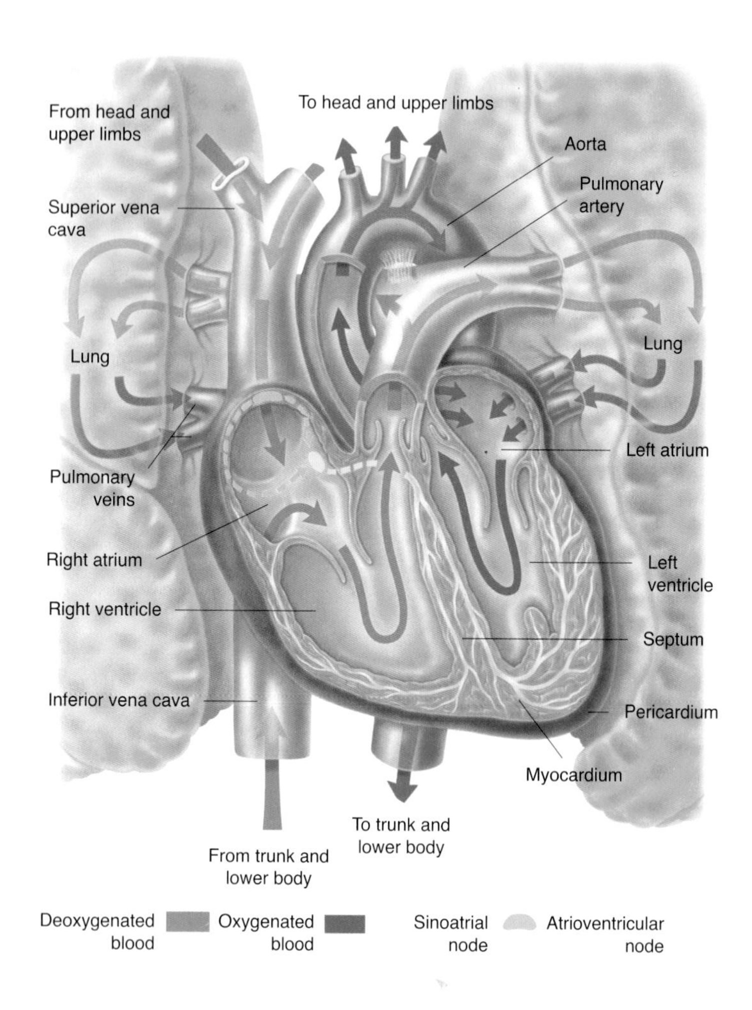

Internal anatomy of the heart.

The circulatory system works on very simple principles: the arteries carry blood away from the heart, and the veins carry blood back to the heart. The heart pumps blood directly into very large arteries, which keep dividing into slightly smaller arteries as they get further

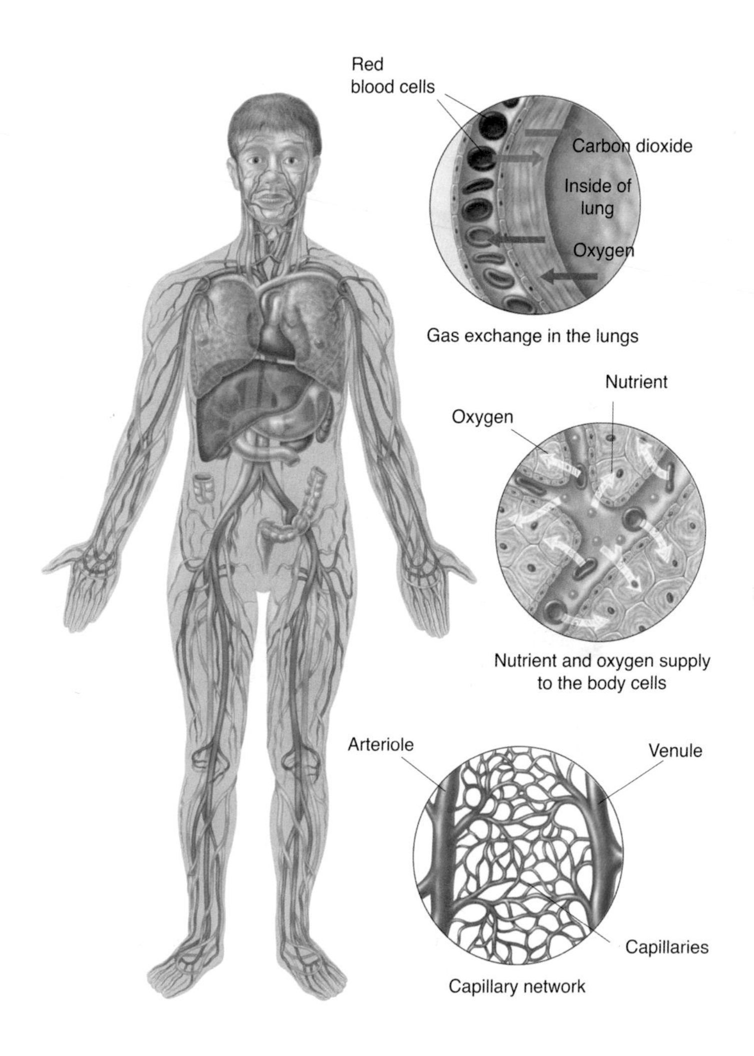

Circulatory system.

from the heart. Eventually, they become tiny as they reach the individual cells, and form part of what is called a capillary. The capillaries surround all the cells in the body, and are made up of an arterial supply and a venous drainage. The veins that form a capillary are tiny to start with, but as they drain back towards the heart, they get bigger and bigger as they join together, until they become the huge central veins that drain directly into the heart.

All cells in the body need to be supplied with oxygen and nutrients, including the cells that form the heart muscle. The blood vessels that supply this muscle are the coronary arteries, and they come off the aorta just after it leaves the heart. There are two main coronary arteries, called the left and the right, but like all other arteries in the body, they divide into several smaller branches.

There are four valves in the heart. Each atrium is divided from the ventricle on the same side by a valve, and each ventricle is divided from its main arterial trunk by a valve. They are named according to the chart on page 7.

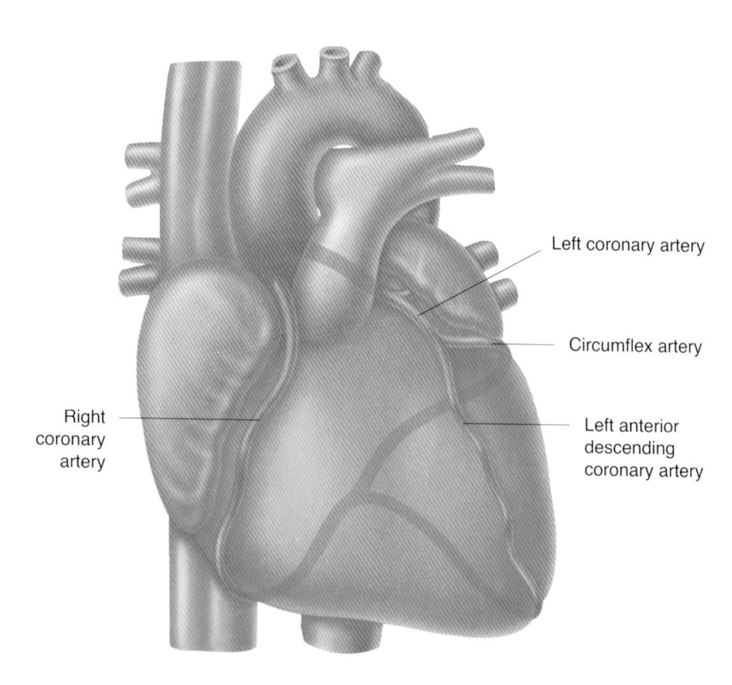

Anatomy of the coronary arteries.

THE HEART VALVES

Name of valve	Side	Separating
Mitral	Left	Atrium and ventricle
Aortic	Left	Ventricle and aorta
Tricuspid	Right	Atrium and ventricle
Pulmonary	Right	Ventricle and pulmonary artery

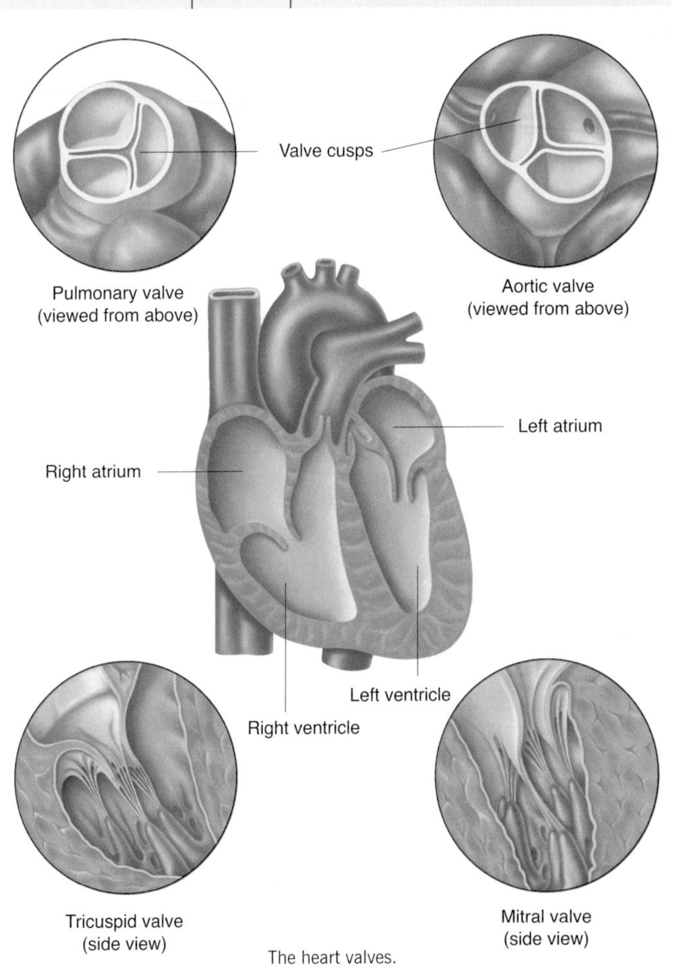

The heart valves.

The heart valves only allow blood to flow in one direction. The mitral and tricuspid valves allow blood to flow from atrium to ventricle, and the aortic and pulmonary valves allow blood to flow from ventricle to arterial trunk. This, in combination with the rhythmic pumping of the heart, facilitates one-way flow around the circulation.

Each valve is made up of either two or three leaflets, which are thin, membranous structures rather like parachutes. The mitral and tricuspid valves are attached to the wall of the ventricle that they serve by tendinous strands called chordae tendinae, similar to parachute lines. These prevent the leaflets billowing into the atrium when the ventricle pumps.

As we shall see later, problems with both the coronary arteries and the valves affect the function of the heart, and in many cases this can be remedied by surgery.

How the heart works

In order to pump blood efficiently around the body, the heart needs to beat at an adequate frequency (heart rate, HR), and with each beat it needs to pump out an adequate quantity of blood (stroke volume, SV). The efficiency of the heart can be measured as a number (cardiac output, CO). The cardiac output can

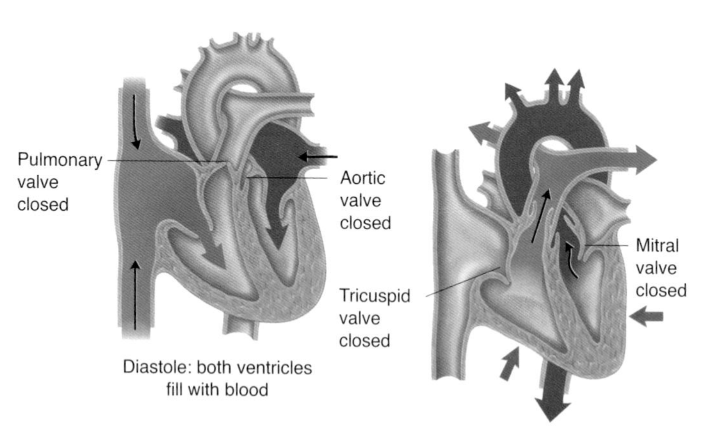

Rhythm of the heart.

be calculated from the heart rate and stroke volume using a simple formula:

CO	=	HR	x	SV
Cardiac output		Heart rate		Stroke volume

From this, you can see that anything that reduces either the heart rate or the stroke volume can lower the cardiac output. The body tries to compensate for such eventualities, and if, for example, the heart rate drops, the stroke volume will automatically increase to give the same overall cardiac output. However, this compensation has a limit, above which the cardiac output will start to fall, and symptoms will start to appear, such as breathlessness and ankle swelling.

The heart rate is dependent upon an inbuilt pacemaker in the wall of the right atrium. In the average person, this beats about 72 times per minute. During exercise, when a higher cardiac output is required by the body, it can increase up to about 200 times per minute. The stroke volume is dependent upon the muscle of the ventricular wall, and its ability to contract or squeeze. In the normal person, it is about 70 millilitres of blood per beat.

From the above equation, you can work out that the average cardiac output is:

HR	x	SV	=	CO
72	x	70	=	5.04
beats per minute		millilitres per beat		litres per minute

If the ventricle is damaged in any way, such as after a heart attack, the stroke volume may be reduced accordingly, and the heart may automatically speed up to compensate.

The blood pressure can be calculated from the cardiac output and the resistance in the blood vessels around the body. It represents the pressure of blood in the arteries, and can be measured directly by applying a pressurised cuff to your arm (called a sphygmomanometer).

Blood pressure is expressed as two numbers, and measured in millimetres of mercury (mmHg):

$$\frac{X}{Y}$$

where X is called the systolic pressure, and Y is called the diastolic pressure.

When the heart actually beats and pumps blood into the arteries, it is called the systolic phase, and after every beat it relaxes to refill the ventricles, which is the diastolic phase. The normal blood pressure is about:

$$\frac{120}{80} \text{ mmHg}$$

The blood pressure can be affected by many things, as we shall see later, and is also a risk factor for various forms of heart disease.

KEY POINTS

- ✓ The heart consists of four chambers
- ✓ Arteries take blood away from the heart, and veins take blood back to the heart
- ✓ There are four valves in the heart allowing one-way blood flow
- ✓ The heart rate relies on an in-built pacemaker

Ischaemic heart disease

Ischaemic heart disease (IHD) is the disease process that causes angina and heart attacks. The word 'ischaemic' simply means reduction in blood supply, which is what happens to the heart muscle when the coronary arteries narrow. IHD is the biggest single cause of death in the United Kingdom, killing nearly 250,000 people every year. The UK has one of the highest death rates in the world from this condition.

Fortunately, there have been many recent advances in both primary prevention of IHD, and the treatment of existing disease by drugs and non-surgical intervention. The resulting effect is that fewer people should require surgery for this condition in the future.

What goes wrong

Most people who need heart surgery have ischaemic heart disease that has developed as a result of atherosclerosis, which causes narrowing of the coronary arteries. This process is often referred to as 'furring up' of the arteries in an analogy to the way water pipes fur up. You will often hear doctors refer to the narrowing as a 'stenosis'. It is a slow, progressive process, whereby fatty deposits build up on the inner wall of the arteries. As these deposits (or 'plaques') enlarge, the artery narrows, and the normally smooth inner wall is also disrupted. This disruption, as well as the tendency of the plaques to crack, can cause a blood clot (thrombosis) to form.

Usually, atherosclerosis develops slowly over many years without causing any symptoms, but there are several things that may speed up the process. If a thrombosis occurs, it usually causes a sudden complete blockage of an already narrowed artery, and the person has an acute heart attack, also called a myocardial infarction (MI). You will find a more detailed explanation of

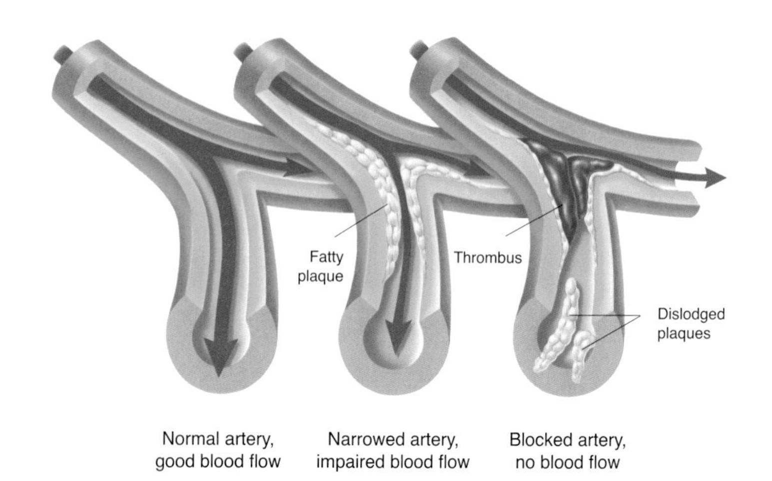

Atherosclerosis.

all this in the Family Doctor publication *Understanding Coronary Heart Disease*.

Exactly what symptoms any one person experiences will depend to an extent on the effects of the atherosclerotic disease, but they can be very variable in any case. The narrowing in the artery may be able to supply the volume of blood required by the heart muscles (ventricles) at rest.

However, during exercise, when the heart needs extra oxygen to fuel the extra work that it has to do, the narrowing may not allow enough blood to get through. This creates an area of heart muscle beyond the narrowing that can't work as efficiently because it is starved of oxygen. This is known as an ischaemic area.

The effects of oxygen shortage on the heart are similar to those of muscular cramp, which is also the result of a muscle getting insufficient oxygen. In this case, the pain takes the form of angina and results from oxygen starvation of the myocardial cells. As with cramp, oxygen starvation also affects the muscle's ability to continue working, but how much the heart muscle function is reduced will depend on which part of the artery is narrowed and in how many places. If there is only one narrowing, and it is quite a long way down the coronary artery, then only a very small part of the heart will be affected, and there will be very little noticeable effect overall.

On the other hand, if there are several narrowings, and they are much nearer the beginning (or origin) of the coronary arteries, then a much larger area of heart muscle will be affected, and the person will be much more likely to get symptoms.

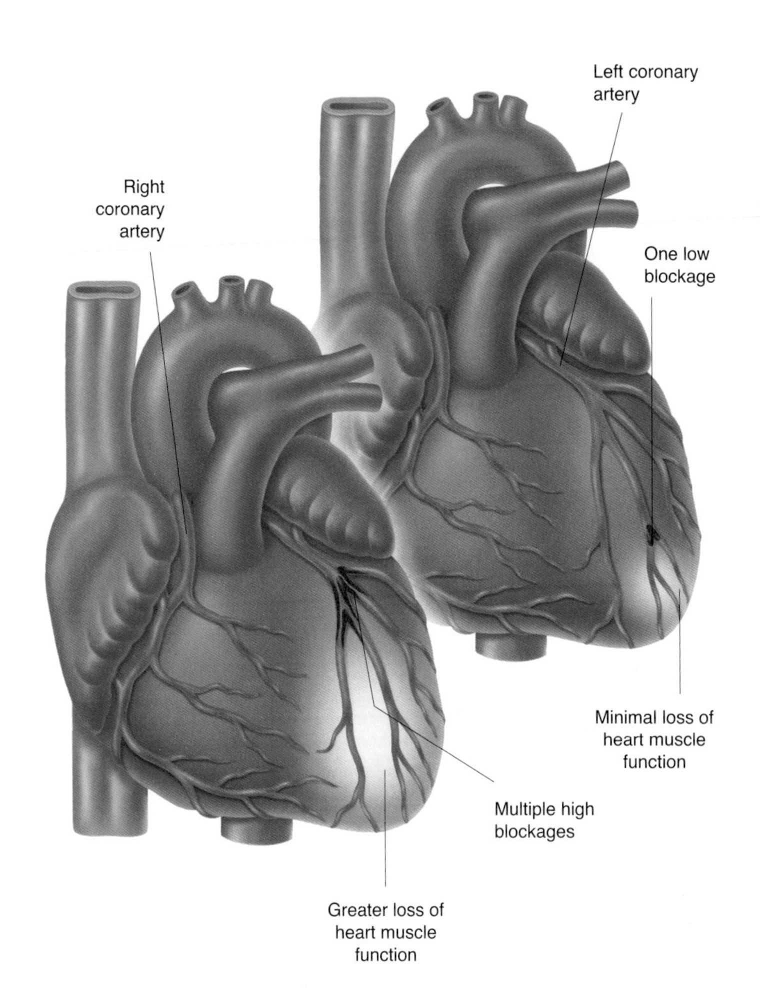

Stages leading to heart failure.

Narrowing near the origin of the vessel is known as proximal disease, and is much more common than narrowing near the end (distal disease). Proximal disease is obviously much more serious in its implications, particularly when it affects the very beginning of the left coronary artery, called the left main stem. If the left main stem blocks off, sudden death is almost certain because the main part of the heart will be starved of blood. For this reason, people who have been shown to have a tight narrowing of the left main stem are often kept in hospital for an operation on the next available operating list. Even in the absence of symptoms, it is serious enough to require urgent surgery, and it is not safe to put such patients on a routine waiting list.

The nature and seriousness of a person's symptoms are related to the amount of muscle function that has been lost. They might include angina, a heart attack and/or heart failure, depending on the degree of damage. Again, all this is explained in more detail in the Family Doctor publication *Understanding Coronary Heart Disease*.

KEY POINTS

- ✓ Ischaemic heart disease (IHD) is caused by atherosclerosis
- ✓ Chest pain (angina) is the main symptom

Valvular heart disease

The purpose of a heart valve is to allow blood to flow in one direction only between two distinct parts of the heart and the circulation. Normally, this means that it will let blood into a chamber or major vessel, but won't let it back out the way it came in.

There are two broad ways in which a heart valve can become damaged:

- It can become narrowed (stenosis), so not enough blood can be pushed through the gap with each stroke of the heart; the heart tries to pump harder, putting it under extra strain.
- It can become leaky or incompetent (regurgitation). In this case, some blood will flow back into the chamber that it came from, so, again, the heart

Normal valves

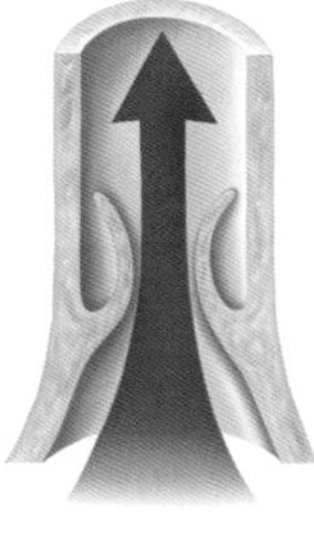

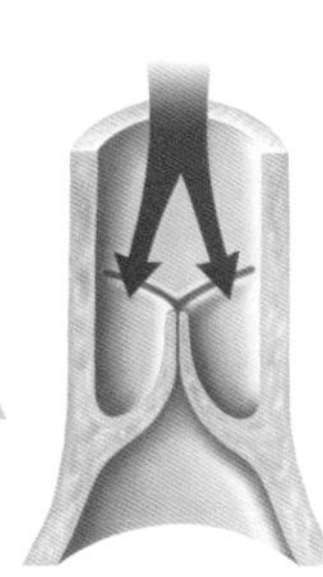

Diseased valves

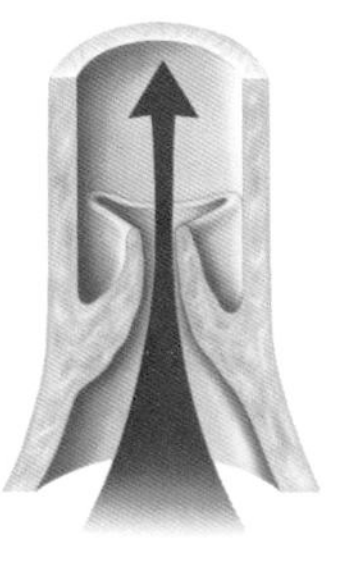

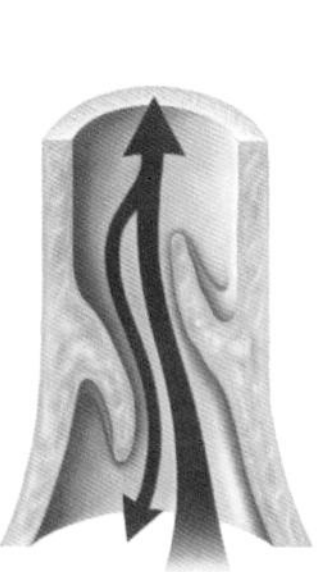

Valve problems.

needs to work harder to pump enough blood out in the right direction.

In both of these conditions the heart has to work harder, as mentioned above. The consequence of the heart working harder is that it becomes bigger and bulkier, much like any over-exercised muscle. There is, however, a limit to how big the heart can become. Once the limit is reached, and if nothing has been done to treat the underlying condition, the heart will start to fail.

The medical term for the bigger, bulkier heart is 'cardiac hypertrophy'. A large number of patients undergoing heart surgery have hypertrophy, but far fewer have hearts that have actually gone into failure. The risks of surgery are much higher for a patient in heart failure, so the timing of referral for surgery is crucial.

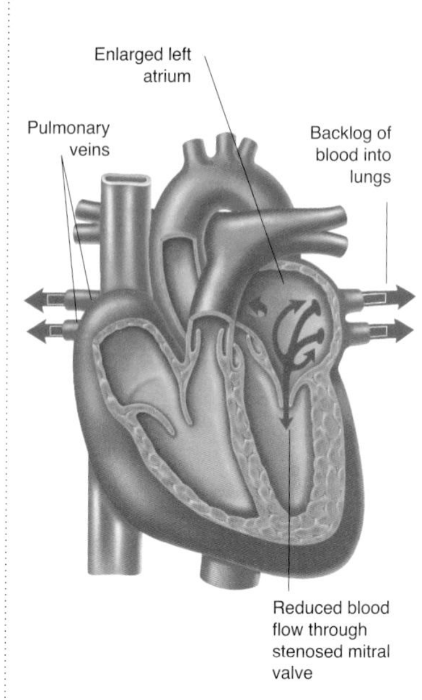

Mitral stenosis.

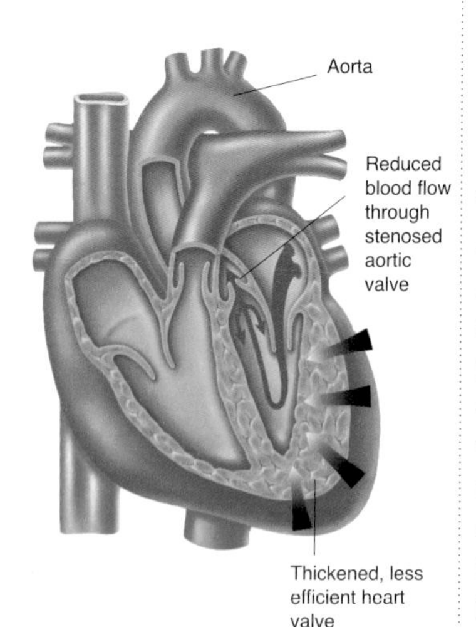

Aortic stenosis.

WHAT GOES WRONG

There are a large number of causes of valvular heart disease (VHD), some of which can cause either stenosis or regurgitation. Any of the four heart valves may become diseased, but the mitral or aortic valves are most often affected, and over 99 per cent of heart valve operations are on one or other of these. This is because they are both in the left side of the heart which is exposed to much higher pressures and stresses than the right side.

Some individuals may have a combination of valve diseases, for example, combined aortic stenosis and regurgitation is known as 'mixed aortic valve disease'. Similarly, both aortic and mitral valves can be affected by disease in one person, and this is especially common when the cause is rheumatic fever.

The effects of valvular heart disease can range from easily tolerated to profoundly disabling. As we have seen, the underlying process continues to the point where the heart cannot cope any more and starts to fail, usually giving the initial symptoms of breathlessness and angina. After these symptoms, caused by left-sided heart failure, the right side may start to fail. Among other things, this will cause swollen ankles and legs, resulting from the backlog of blood trying to return to the heart from the rest of the body.

There is only so much that the heart can put up with and, unless something is done to relieve the strain on it, your condition will rapidly worsen. It is therefore important to recognise when you're starting to get symptoms and to seek specialist help accordingly.

KEY POINTS

- ✓ Valves can become narrowed or leaky
- ✓ Shortness of breath is a common symptom of valve disease

Diagnosis of heart disease

If you do have a heart problem, you will find yourself seeing your general practitioner (GP) at some stage, usually when symptoms appear. A consultation with him or her, and perhaps some tests, will often give the diagnosis. You will probably be referred to a cardiologist at your local hospital.

A cardiologist is a heart specialist but should not be confused with a cardiac surgeon. The cardiologist is the first person to whom you will be referred if you get diagnosed with suspected heart disease. He or she will perform a number of tests to aid in the diagnosis, and may start any combination of a number of different treatments. These are dealt with in the Family Doctor book *Understanding Coronary Heart Disease*. In most cases some medical treatment, such as drugs, will be enough to keep the symptoms at bay for the time being. However, the processes that cause the disease are usually ongoing or progressive, and different drugs may need to be added in increasing doses. It is usually only if these treatments reach a maximum level or fail to control the symptoms that the cardiologist will then refer you to a cardiac surgeon for an opinion about the potential benefits of surgery. Most patients with heart problems, therefore, will never get to meet a cardiac surgeon. This is a very specialised field of medicine and there may not be one in your local hospital. In this event, you will go to see the surgeon at the nearest large centre for cardiac surgery. The cardiologist and the cardiac surgeon will then discuss you and your problems, and decide whether an operation would help, or whether a different option may be better for you.

From the moment you first bring your problem to the attention of your GP (or any doctor), a series of things will happen to you in order

DIAGNOSING HEART DISEASE	
Ischaemic heart disease (IHD)	**Valvular heart disease (VHD)**
History	History
Examination	Examination
Chest X-ray	Chest X-ray
Electrocardiography (ECG)	Electrocardiography (ECG)
Exercise test	Echocardiography
Angiography	Angiography
Blood tests	Blood tests

to establish the diagnosis, as shown in the box above.

History

First of all, your doctor will ask you for a full and detailed description about yourself, both in relation to this particular illness and your symptoms and in relation to other details that may seem unrelated. All this information will be written down in your medical notes, and is known as your 'history'.

It is important for the history to paint as complete a picture as possible, because many little things that might seem unimportant to you may give clues towards your diagnosis. Details about your current problems are usually easy to give, but your past medical history (such as childhood rheumatic fever) and your family history (for example, relatives who have had heart attacks at a young age) are vitally important too.

By the time an accurate history has been taken, before a hand is even laid upon you, a very good idea about your diagnosis has usually been made.

Examination

Next, you will be carefully examined. You may find that your doctor looks at your face, neck, hands and ankles thoroughly, before turning to your chest. This may seem odd, because you have a chest problem, but it is very important, because there are many clues to the diagnosis of heart disease in these areas. He or she may do some other peculiar things when examining your chest, such as tapping with the fingers, which is known as percussion. You will always have your chest listened to

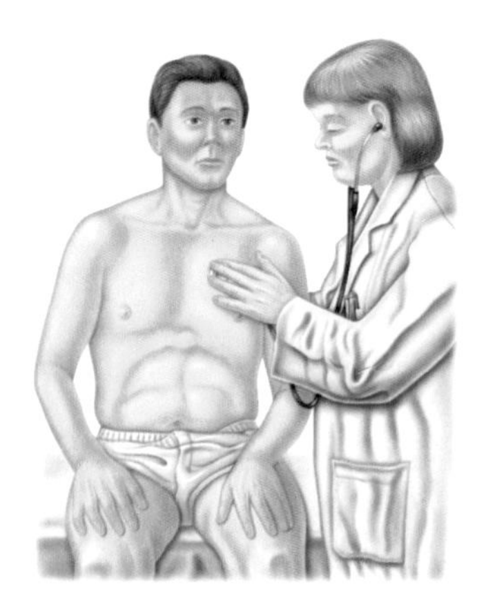

Physical examination.

with a stethoscope, both front and back. Using this, your doctor will be able to listen carefully for any heart murmurs, as well as checking for left heart failure which causes fluid on the lungs.

At this stage, after your history and examination, the diagnosis is pretty clear in the vast majority of cases. Your doctor will then decide, on the basis of his or her suspicions, which tests are needed to confirm this, and which treatment to start.

Chest X-ray

If you have a suspected heart condition, you will almost certainly have a chest X-ray taken at an early stage, although it usually provides only a limited amount of information. If you have IHD, the only findings of interest may be an enlarged heart shadow, and some fluid on the lungs (left heart failure), but you may not have either. Equally, if you have VHD, the findings may be very similar. The

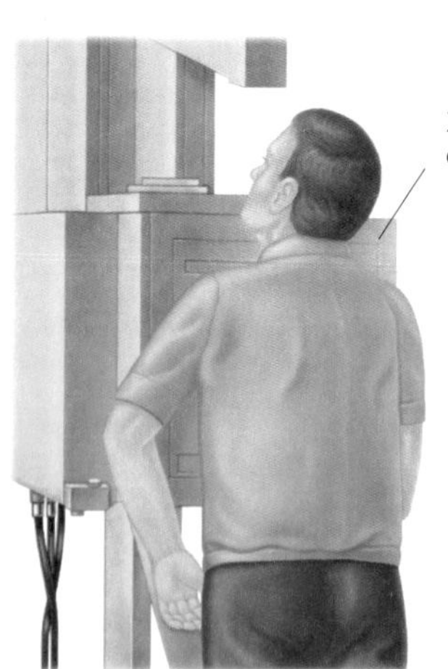

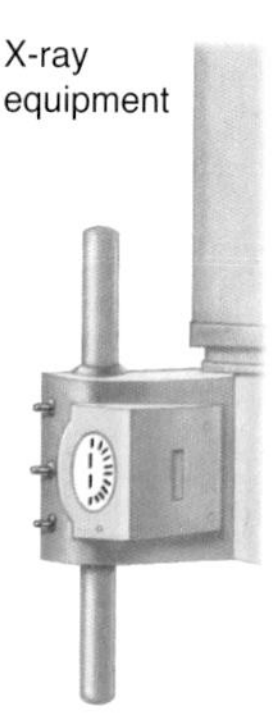

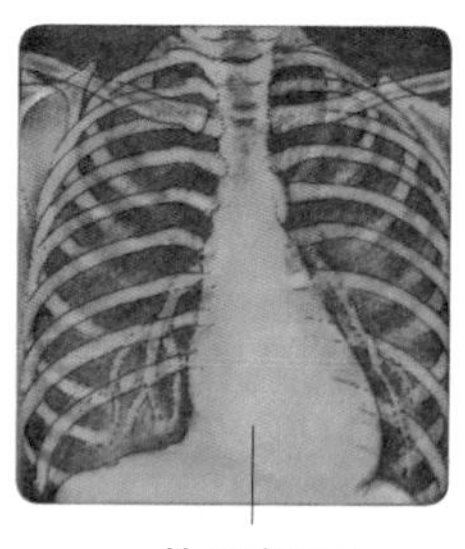

Chest X-ray.

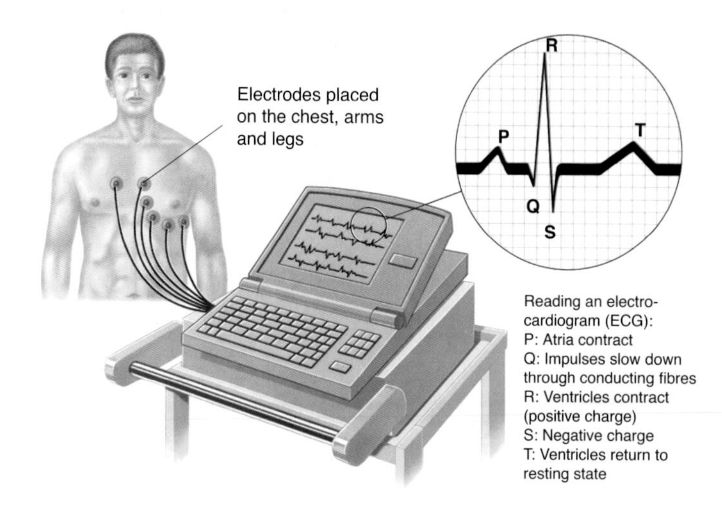

Electrocardiography (ECG).

main importance of a chest X-ray is probably in the elimination of other, more serious disease in the chest.

Electrocardiography electrocardiogram (ECG)

Most people with heart disease will have an ECG performed. It is an electrical tracing of the heart's activity, and gives important information about most of the conditions that affect it.

It is completely painless, and simply involves you lying down and having about ten sticky patches put on your chest, arms and legs. These

WHAT THE ECG CAN REVEAL

- Rhythm abnormalities (such as irregular heart beat)
- Rate abnormalities (too fast or slow)
- Myocardial infarct (recent)
- Myocardial infarct (old)
- Angina
- Enlarged heart (under strain)
- Some valve diseases

are attached by wires to the ECG machine, which records the activity of the heart on a piece of special graph paper. The whole thing takes a couple of minutes.

The doctor looking after you will be interested in your ECG for two reasons: first, to see if there are any abnormalities which may confirm the diagnosis and, second, to compare it with any previous ECGs that you may have had taken, to see if there has been any change in your condition. Important information that can be obtained from the ECG is shown in the box on page 21.

Exercise test

Angina will usually first show itself when you are under stress or exertion. As the condition worsens, it may start to occur at rest. The change indicates a progressive narrowing of the coronary arteries. If you have angina, one of the first tests that you will undergo is the exercise test, or 'stress test'. This takes the form of a continuous ECG recording while you are walking on a treadmill.

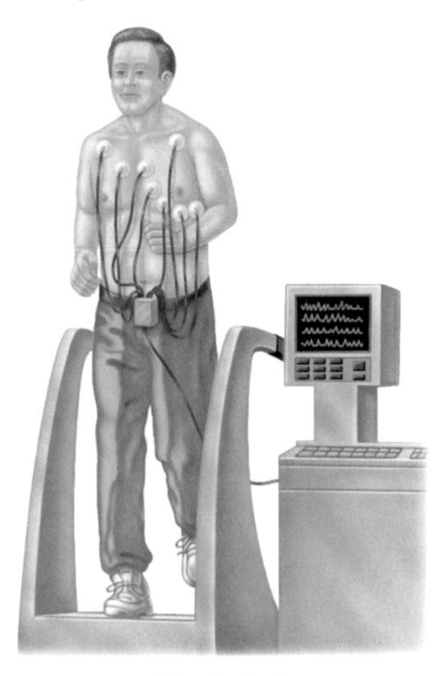

Exercise test.

The wires are attached to you in exactly the same way as for a normal ECG, and the treadmill is started. It starts slowly, and will become a little faster and steeper every 3 minutes. The whole test consists of seven 3-minute periods, but it is not necessary to finish it. You can stop at any time, but the usual reasons are chest pain, shortness of breath or tiredness. A doctor will be watching the ECG tracing on a screen while you perform the test, and may ask you to stop because of changes that he sees, even if you feel fine.

You either 'pass' or 'fail' an exercise test. Passing means that you reach a reasonable level of exercise for your age and ability. Failing means that you develop chest pain, rhythm disturbances, low blood pressure or ECG changes noted by the doctor watching you.

Failing an exercise test is also known as having a 'positive' or 'strongly positive' result. In most cases this will mean that your cardiologist will recommend that you have another procedure called angiography performed (see later).

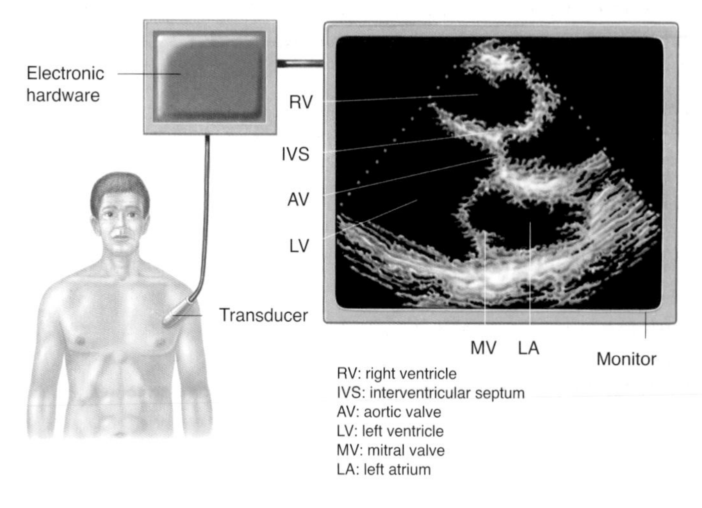

Echocardiography.

Echocardiography

Known as an 'echo' this is another painless and easy test to perform, but one that gives very valuable information about your heart. It is particularly useful in VHD, because it gives a two-dimensional moving image of your heart, and can see the chambers and valves. It is simply an ultrasound scan, similar to the ones that most women will have in pregnancy. You will be asked to lie down on a semi-upright couch, and the operator (either a cardiologist or a specialist echocardiographer) will run the probe across your chest, using a little lubricant jelly to help the contact.

The operator moves the probe from place to place to look at different parts of the heart, while watching the screen. The whole echo is recorded on a video tape, so that it can be watched later by other experts if necessary. Using this test, the valves can be measured for the degree of narrowing or leakiness. The function of the ventricles as pumps can also be observed, by watching how well they contract with each beat. Echocardiography is very useful, because it gives a quick, comfortable result and, as the tapes are kept, comparisons can be made of an individual patient over a period of time, to see whether things are worsening.

Most echocardiograms are performed as described above by moving the probe across the front of your chest. This is called a transthoracic echocardiogram (TTE). There is, however, another form of echocardiography that gives a more accurate image and is particularly useful for certain specific conditions. It is called transoesophageal echocardiography (TOE) and is a little more invasive than TTE. It involves swallowing a tube containing the ultrasound probe into your oesophagus (gullet) and down into your stomach. As some people can find this a bit uncomfortable, the procedure is usually performed under some light sedation. TOE is particularly useful during some heart operations, especially valve surgery, and can show both the anatomy and the result of surgery quite clearly.

Angiography

Also known as 'angio' or cardiac catheterisation, this is the definitive test for looking at coronary artery disease (IHD). You will be required to have angiography if there is a strong suspicion that something other than drug treatment needs to be done to your coronary arteries to make you better. This suspicion is raised if you 'fail' your exercise test, or sometimes if you continue to get angina after a heart attack.

Unlike the previous tests, it involves a drip being put in your arm, and you'll be given a mild sedative to relax you, although you'll remain conscious during the procedure. This test takes place in a special room or 'suite' called the 'Cath Lab', with a movable bed for

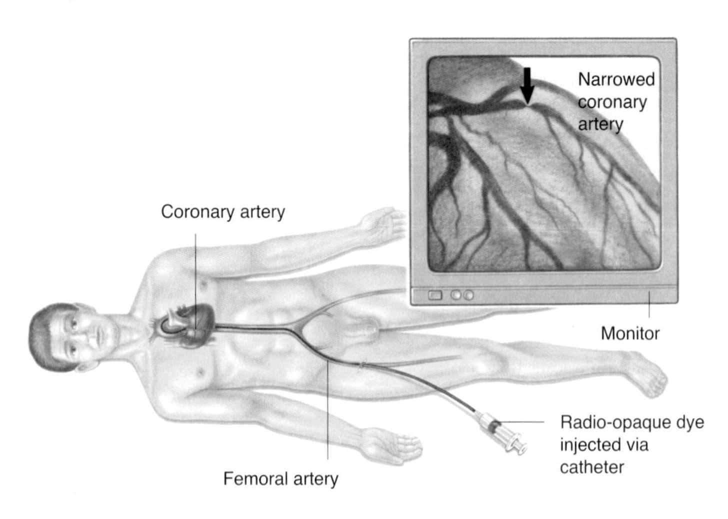

Angiography.

you to lie on, and a big overhead X-ray machine. The actual procedure needs a larger drip to be placed in one of the large arteries in your arm or leg. This is usually in your groin or in front of your elbow, and is performed under local anaesthetic. Some dye is then injected down this big drip, and passes into your heart and your coronary arteries. The procedure is being filmed the whole time by the X-ray machine. By injecting dye down each of the coronary arteries in turn, it is easy to identify where the narrowings are, and how severe they are. It ends up giving a sort of 'road-map' of the heart. Dye can also be used to show how efficiently the heart is working as a pump, and information may also be gained about the condition of the heart valves and the size of the aorta.

The whole procedure takes about half an hour, and you can go home after a rest of about four hours. The film is then looked at by your cardiologist and, if necessary, by the cardiac surgeon.

Other tests

There are a number of other tests and investigations that are used to diagnose heart disease. Some of these are simple and common, and some of them are more complex and only used in specific circumstances. Of these, you are most likely to have blood tests at some stage. Those that may provide information, which may be significant in terms of the heart disease itself, are for cholesterol (and triglyceride) levels and cardiac enzymes.

If you are suspected of having IHD, particularly if you have a family history of it, your doctor will measure your cholesterol levels and, if they are high, you will be given advice and possibly some treatment. Failure to recognise and treat this will result in more rapid progression of the coronary artery narrowings.

Cardiac enzymes are measured if you have had an acute myocardial infarction (MI or heart attack), or even a bad attack of angina. You get very high levels in the blood if you have had a heart attack, but much lower levels with angina. They are therefore helpful in the differentiation between the two, and will guide appropriate treatment for whichever is diagnosed.

There are a number of other tests used in the diagnosis of heart disease. These include thallium, MUGA (multi-gated acquisition), and PET (positron emission tomography) scans. These are procedures that involve the use of radioactively labelled compounds or isotopes, and they are performed in a Department of Nuclear Medicine on a 'day visit' basis. If you are having one of these tests, you will have an injection of a tiny dose of a radioactive marker, and then you will be screened by a special machine. There is nothing dangerous or uncomfortable about either of these tests. They do not make a diagnosis of the specific disease process, but aid in giving information about the heart's pump function, and the general state of the heart muscle.

In addition there is increasing use of cardiac MRI (magnetic resonance imaging), as well as a form of echocardiography carried out under higher work conditions, known as 'stress echo' or 'dobutamine echo' because of the drug used. More about these and other diagnostic tests can be found in other books in the Family Doctor series.

KEY POINTS

- ✓ The diagnosis can usually be made easily
- ✓ There are many tests to confirm the diagnosis

Non-surgical treatment

You will not usually be considered for an operation until all other options have been exhausted. This is reasonable, because a heart operation is a large undertaking, with risks involved, and should be avoided if possible. In most cases, you will be receiving some form of drug therapy for your heart complaint, well before surgery is considered. This is often altered or the doses increased according to your symptoms, and is prescribed either by your GP or by your cardiologist at the clinic. There are many drugs available that act to help the heart, and you often need to be on a combination of them, because they work in different ways.

Apart from drugs, there are several other forms of treatment for heart disease that can be considered either before or instead of surgery:

- Angioplasty (PTCA)
- Stenting
- Balloon valvuloplasty
- Pacemaker insertion
- Defibrillator insertion
- Other treatments for abnormal rhythms.

These are often performed, but sometimes work for only a limited period of time and, if the symptoms return, you may well need an operation anyway.

Sometimes, however, the investigations reveal that the disease process is severe enough to warrant surgery, and there is no real point in considering other courses of treatment. The best form of treatment for you is normally decided upon by your cardiologist. When he or she thinks that it is time for surgery to be considered as an option, you will be referred for a consultation with a cardiac surgeon at your nearest cardiothoracic centre. The fact that you are referred for a consultation does not necessarily mean that you definitely need an operation.

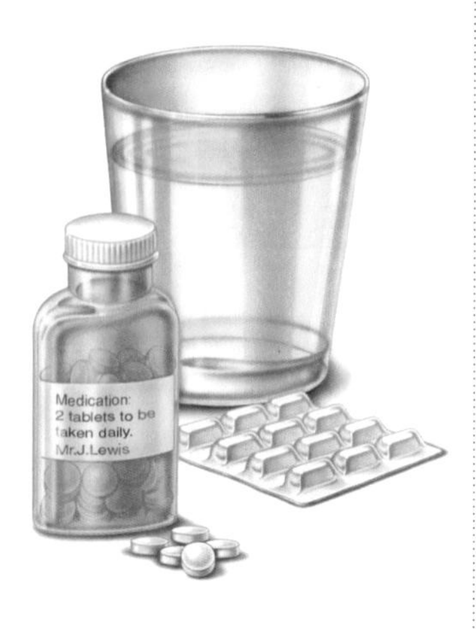

However, it means that you will be able to discuss the risks and benefits of surgery with the surgeon, and in most cases an operation will follow.

Drug therapy

This is a very complex subject, with a huge number of drugs on the market today, and it is not necessary to explain how they all work. If you would like to find out more about drug treatments, there are detailed explanations in the Family Doctor publication *Understanding Heart Failure.*

Ischaemic heart disease (IHD)

If you have angina, it is very likely that you will have some form of nitrate therapy. You may be on a regular dose of ISMN or ISDN, but you will almost certainly have GTN (glyceryl trinitrate) to take during acute attacks. GTN relaxes the muscle in your blood vessels, allowing them to expand or dilate. Your GTN will either come as tablets or a spray, both of which are for use under your tongue, or come as a patch to place on your skin. GTN will relieve your angina attack, but may leave you flushed or with a headache.

Beta blockers are also commonly used in IHD, because they reduce the blood pressure, slow the heart, and reduce the work that the heart has to do. This means that the energy (and thus oxygen) requirement is less, so they should reduce your symptoms of angina.

Calcium antagonists are the third main group of drugs used in IHD. Among other effects, they allow your coronary arteries to dilate, thus allowing more blood through the narrowings.

These three groups of drugs comprise the maximum drug therapy for IHD. If you are taking all three, you are receiving what is known as 'triple therapy', and if you continue to get symptoms you will probably require an operation, or perhaps one of the alternative treatments mentioned below. It is quite common to be on other heart drugs when you have IHD, and now there are a number of new and very effective treatments. You may also be on other drugs that do not specifically work on the IHD, but on associated problems such as heart failure or a coincidental irregular heart rhythm.

Valvular heart disease (VHD)

Most symptoms related to VHD result from heart failure which causes fluid retention. Diuretics (water tablets) are very useful, because they make you pass urine, and this gets rid of unnessary fluid that you have in your body. This is a great help in decreasing both your breathlessness, and the swelling in your legs and ankles.

ACE (angiotensin-converting enzyme) inhibitors help in heart failure, by dilating some of the blood vessels coming into the heart, therefore easing some of the strain of pumping. Digoxin has been very valuable in heart failure for a long time, particularly if you have a fast, irregular heart beat. It slows the heart rate and increases the efficiency of the pump. It is, however, gradually losing favour as a first-line drug for heart failure as new generations of cardiac drugs are being developed.

ANGIOPLASTY AND STENTING

In certain instances, you may have been investigated for IHD, and your angiogram will show either a single narrowing in a single coronary artery, or perhaps single narrowings in only two of the arteries. In such cases, there are clever ways of getting rid of the narrowings

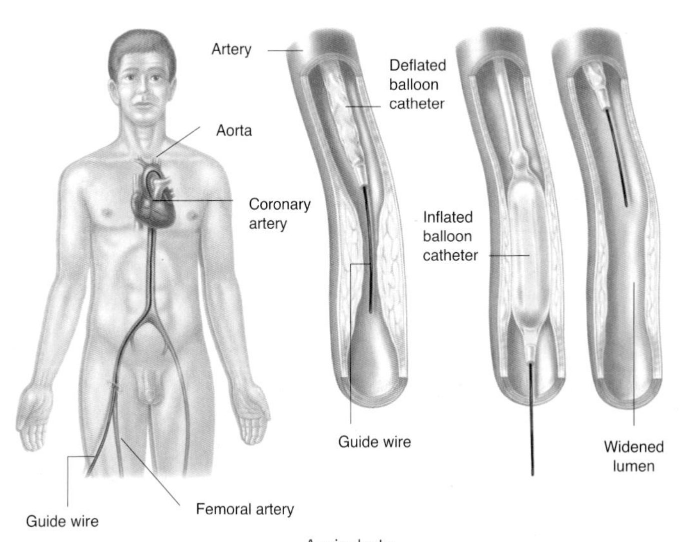

Angioplasty.

without the need for an operation. Precisely which individuals can benefit from these procedures is not always easy to decide, and there is a lot of research looking into this. Having said that, however, they can still be a useful addition to the other forms of treatment available.

Angioplasty, also known as PTCA (percutaneous transcoronary angioplasty), was first performed in 1977, and is a safe and extremely common procedure nowadays. It involves the same preparation as for an angiogram (see page 24), with a catheter being passed into an artery in the arm or groin. Under X-ray control using dye, a wire is passed across the narrowing in the coronary artery. The wire used is different in that it has a deflated 'sausage-shaped' balloon on the end. When the part of the wire with the balloon on is lying across the narrowing, it is inflated, which compresses the blockage and leaves the artery open again.

The advantages of this technique are that it can be done without a general anaesthetic, is relatively quick, and does not usually involve a hospital stay of more than one night. The disadvantages are that there is a chance of the blood vessel narrowing again and the angina reappearing. If this happens, you can either have the angioplasty repeated or have an operation. This decision will largely be up to your cardiologist who will have to assess whether this is the right treatment for you. The decision depends on the length and number of narrowings.

Everyone who is about to have angioplasty needs to understand that there is the possibility of completely blocking the coronary artery during the procedure. This shows up as changes on the ECG monitor, and the patient may experience some chest pain. If this happens, an urgent bypass operation is needed. This must be performed immediately, so all patients who undergo angioplasty must sign a consent form for a bypass operation as well, just in case it should be necessary. The chances of this happening are small, however, and are only about 1–2 per cent.

Stenting is very similar to angioplasty, in that it is performed in the angiography laboratory under local anaesthetic and mild sedation only. The difference with stenting is that the balloon is surrounded by a piece of collapsed wire mesh (stent). When the balloon is inflated, the mesh expands to a fixed and open position, which should help prevent the vessel narrowing again in the future (see figure on page 31). The balloon catheter is then removed, leaving the stent in place. The chances of this working are slightly better than angioplasty, with less

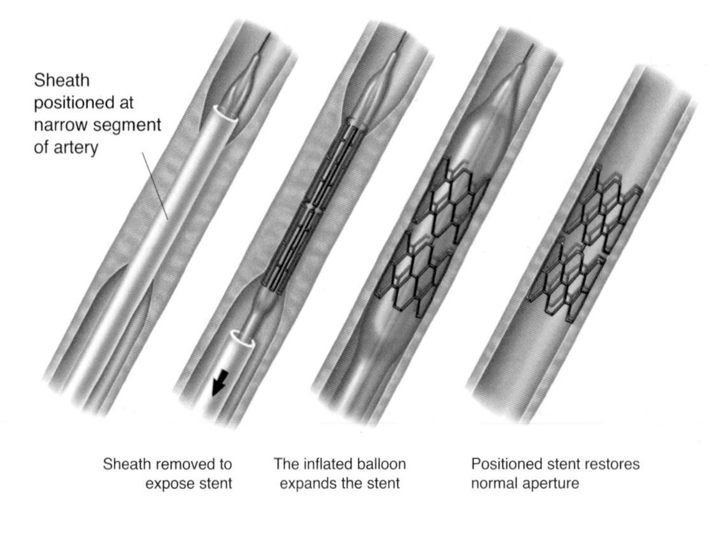

Stenting.

than 20 per cent getting symptoms again within six months.

Stenting is now standard practice in PTCA and it is almost unknown to have a balloon angioplasty performed without stent insertion. It combines the active process of opening up the narrowing with a support mechanism to make sure that the artery remains open for as long as possible. There is a wide variety of different stents available, each with its own proposed advantages. Stents are the subject of a great deal of research at present, and to date it has been shown that they significantly reduce the chances of the arteries re-narrowing. There are a number of new generations of stents now available, each with their own purported advantages. Some of these can slowly leak out beneficial drugs after implantation (drug-eluting stents), and are expected to be associated with very good results in the future.

It has also been shown that, in some cases, they may offer a similar outcome to a triple bypass, but without all the risks associated with having a major heart operation.

Balloon valvuloplasty

This is a relatively uncommon procedure, but still has a place in the treatment of stenotic (narrowed) valve disease. It is performed in the angiography laboratory under mild sedation, and involves a balloon catheter being passed across a narrowed heart valve and inflated, in much the same way as angioplasty.

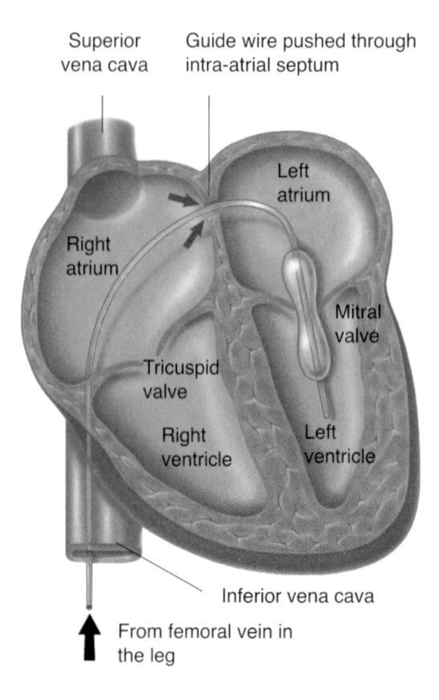

Balloon valvuloplasty.

Over 95 per cent of valvuloplasties in adults are performed for mitral stenosis, but it is also used in some children born with narrow valves.

ELECTROPHYSIOLOGY

Cardiac electrophysiology is a specialised area that deals with rhythm disturbances of the heart. There is a wide variety of investigations and treatments available, including a number of very recent advances. The treatments are not surgical but are usually performed in a specifically designated area or even in the angiography laboratory. Common treatments include pacemaker and defibrillator insertion, but more complex procedures are becoming increasingly used. Rhythm problems can be cured by procedures such as nodal ablation and pulmonary vein isolation, which can be carried out without the need for a general anaesthetic. The Prime Minister, Tony Blair, recently had such a procedure performed successfully for a rhythm disturbance.

KEY POINTS

- ✓ Operations are avoided if possible
- ✓ There are many drugs and other treatments to be tried before surgery

Heart surgery

RISKS AND BENEFITS

The whole point of having a heart operation is to get rid of your symptoms and to increase your life expectancy. It is a major undertaking, but is becoming increasingly safe nowadays as research and technology move forward. Most cardiothoracic centres in this country perform between four and ten heart operations every day. This means that over 30,000 people have heart surgery in this country every year.

For most of these people, it puts an end to their symptoms, whether angina or breathlessness, and brings a vast improvement in their quality of life, and in many cases a complete return to normal. Ask anybody who used to get angina what it feels like to be free from it again, and you will have an idea of the kind of relief surgery can offer. It appears to be really easy these days, because most people whose cases are straightforward go home about five or six days after their operation. Nevertheless, heart surgery is still a major operation, however skilled or advanced we become at it, and it is important that, for all its benefits, the potential risks are taken seriously.

When you are going to have a heart operation, your surgeon will discuss the risks with you, usually at the clinic when you first see him or her, and again the day before the operation. You will be asked to sign a consent form during one of these visits. This is a declaration by you that you understand the nature of the operation, and the risks of death and other complications associated with it.

It is very important that you and your family understand the risks involved when you sign the consent form. Doctors talk about risk in terms of the chances of death during the operation, and the chances of developing a serious complication such as a stroke. There are, of course, a great number of potential complications but most of these are minor, such as wound infections, chest infections and constipation. The major complications such as stroke and temporary kidney failure are always discussed in detail with the patient.

The two main factors that contribute to the risk of your operation are the type of operation itself, and your health before the operation. Obviously some operations take longer than others, and some are more complicated than others. In general, the longer and more complex your operation, the greater the risk.

More importantly, the health of the patient before the operation must be carefully considered. Someone who has no other medical problems, apart from that for which they are having the operation, would be considered 'low risk'. On the other hand, if you have other serious medical problems, such as lung disease or kidney disease, your risks are going to be higher. The condition of your heart also needs to be taken into consideration. If you have never had a heart attack, and it is working well as a pump, you are at lower risk than somebody who may have some scarred areas of muscle from heart attacks and whose heart is less efficient.

The surgeon will take these things and many other factors, such as your age and whether you still smoke, into consideration, and calculate a percentage risk for you personally, for both death and serious complications. The figure quoted is carefully calculated for each individual patient according to a large number of different features. He or she will tell you this figure and explain why before you sign the consent form. For most patients undergoing heart surgery the risk of both of these tragic eventualities is between two and three per cent.

Heart surgery is offered to patients for one (or both) of two main reasons: these are for symptomatic benefit or prognostic benefit. Symptomatic benefit is very easy to understand, and applies to people who get severe angina or breathlessness despite maximal drug therapy. It is all related to quality of life and, if you find that the kind of life that you would like to lead is severely restricted, the chances are that you should undertake the risks of surgery. If you are offered prognostic benefit, it means that your chances of living longer are better with surgery than without it, and are usually related to the severity of the disease as shown on the angiogram.

It is difficult to offer prognostic benefit to patients over the age of 70, because this group are more likely to have unrelated illnesses and disease, which may reduce life expectancy in themselves. Obviously, some patients fall into both categories.

WAITING TIMES AND CANCELLATION

The very nature of cardiac surgery makes it very unpredictable. There are very many 'emergencies', each of which takes up an operating theatre slot, and a bed in the intensive care unit (ICU) or ward. This has two effects on you as the routine waiting-list patient:

- The waiting time that you are given may not be accurate and, even when you get given a date for admission, you may find that when you ring the ward in the morning as instructed there is no bed for you and you can't come in. This can be very frustrating for you, because you may well be frightened or apprehensive about the operation, and have worked yourself up for it. The staff are all aware of this and do not cancel admissions unless it is absolutely necessary, but if emergency cases have taken the beds it cannot be avoided.

- When you have been admitted for your operation, there is still a chance that your operation may be cancelled until another day. Again, this is usually caused by an emergency case taking your operation slot, or sometimes if there are no beds on the ICU. When you have had your operation, you need to go to the ICU, usually for one night. You are usually expected to move back to the ward the following day. This makes a space for the next patient to have his or her operation and go to the ICU. Sometimes, a patient might be a bit slow to wake up, or may need an extra day or so on the ICU. This effectively prevents another person's operation from being performed. Unfortunately, it is impossible to predict who will stay more than one night, but we still need to allocate patients to specific operating lists. This is why there are so many cancellations. If you are cancelled, however, you will not usually be sent home, but be put first on your consultant's next operating list. This may be the next day, but sometimes you might have to wait a little longer. Sadly, there is nothing any of the staff can do to prevent this.

PREPARING FOR SURGERY

Unless you have a particularly complicated problem, which means that you need some specialised investigations as an in-patient, you will normally be admitted to hospital the day before your operation. Some hospitals ask you to attend a pre-admission clinic the week before. Either at this clinic or in hospital the day before your operation, there are a number of routine tests and checks that you will have to go through (see the box). The medications that you are taking will also be checked by the doctor, because there are some that need to be stopped before surgery.

There are not many essentials that you need to bring to hospital with you, but bear in mind that you will be there for about six days, and wardrobe and locker space can be quite limited. Make sure that any pyjamas or other clothes you bring are not too tight fitting, particularly around the neck, because you will have a number of scars and drips.

ROUTINE EVENTS AND CHECKS

- Admission by ward nurse
- History and examination by house officer
- Blood tests (routine)
- ECG
- Chest X-ray
- Visit by ICU nurse
- Consent form
- Visit by surgeon
- Visit by anaesthetist

For women, a supportive, well-fitting cotton bra will help you to be comfortable, even more so if it is one size too big. Apart from your washing kit and something to read, there is nothing else essential. After a couple of days you will be walking around freely, so some casual clothes are useful. These can always be brought in by a friend or relative at that stage.

The ward nurse will familiarise you with the ward environment, and explain to you about shaving your chest for the operation (for a man), and your legs if you are having coronary artery bypass surgery. In some hospitals a member of the nursing staff will actually shave you. Whether it is you or one of the staff, it is important to avoid cuts and abrasions as they are a potential source of infection. He or she will also explain to you about the premedication (pre-med), which is a drug that you are given to relax you about an hour before your operation. Sometimes it takes the form of a tablet, and sometimes a small injection.

You will be seen by a doctor fairly soon after your admission, whose job is to 'clerk you in', and check that everything is as it was when you were seen in clinic. They will also examine you physically to confirm that you are fit for an operation. A word of warning: if you have a cold or flu it is very important that you tell somebody on the ward, either a nurse or a doctor. If you do have either of these conditions, you will have a much higher chance of developing a chest infection while on the ventilator, and so your operation should be cancelled or postponed until your are better.

Routine blood tests, ECG and chest X-ray are performed and checked by one of your doctors to make sure nothing has changed, and you will be asked to sign a consent form after all the details and risks of the operation have been thoroughly explained to you.

You will then be visited by three people who have a key role in your care:

1. The surgeon: he or she will usually come to see you on the evening before your operation to answer any final questions, and to make sure everything is in order.

2. The anaesthetist: he or she is one of the first people you will meet when you arrive in the operating theatre the next day. It is his or her responsibility to see that you are fit for a general anaesthetic.

3. The ICU nurse: when you wake up after your operation, you will be in the ICU. This is a very intimidating environment with lots of people and noises. You will have a tube in your throat helping you breathe, and you will be connected to several drips and machines. The ICU nurse will explain all this, help to reassure you and answer any questions that you may have.

You need to be starved for at least six hours before your operation. If you are going to theatre in the morning, you are simply told not to eat or drink anything from midnight. If your operation is in the afternoon, you are usually allowed a light breakfast. It is vital that you do not break this rule and do not eat or drink anything, because it is dangerous for you, and your operation will have to be cancelled. You are allowed to brush your teeth and have mouth washes, however. People with diabetes will often have a drip put up before the operation, and blood sugar will be carefully monitored by the ward staff during the period of starvation.

The anaesthetic

If you have had an operation before you will know what a general anaesthetic (GA) is. If not, it simply means that you get put to sleep for your operation so you do not feel anything, and then woken up at the end of it. This is performed by a mixture of gases and intravenous drugs, and while you are asleep a machine called a ventilator breathes for you. This is necessary because one of the anaesthetic drugs paralyses all your muscles including the ones that you use to breathe.

When you arrive in the operating department, you will be greeted by a member of the operating team, usually a theatre nurse or operating department practitioner (ODP). This person will welcome you and make you feel comfortable before transferring you to a room adjoining the theatre, called the anaesthetic room. This is where you will meet your anaesthetist again, and where you will be put to sleep for your operation. The theatre nurse or ODP will ask you a number of questions and go through a series of checks to make sure that everything is in order (including checking that you are the right patient!). In this room, you will have two drips put into your arm, one in a vein for the anaesthetic drugs, and one in an artery in your wrist which measures your blood pressure continuously. You will also be attached to an ECG monitor. At this point you are ready to be put to sleep, and the anaesthetist will give you oxygen through a mask for a minute or two. A drug is then injected down through your drip which will make you go to sleep very quickly. It is important to realise that this is the last thing you will remember before you wake up in ICU.

It is important to realise that this is the last thing you will remember before you wake up in ICU

When you are asleep, your muscles are paralysed, so you will be connected to the ventilator which will breathe for you. Before you go into theatre, several other tubes and drips will be put into you, but of course, you will not feel any of this. Among these are a urinary catheter, which is a tube put into your bladder, and a 'central line', which is a drip put into one of the veins in your neck. This is similar to the drip in the vein in your arm, but usually has three or four channels to allow the infusion of several different drugs that you may need during and after surgery. You are now ready for your operation!

Cardiopulmonary bypass

Before it is possible to perform an operation on the heart, several special factors must be taken into account. One is that the heart is a beating organ, and does not stay still, which obviously creates problems in performing delicate surgery. In the 1950s a machine was developed which enabled surgeons to stop the heart and lungs while the operation was being done. It is called the cardiopulmonary bypass machine, and is the main reason why heart surgery has only been possible for such a short period of time compared with other branches of surgery. Although the technology continues to be improved all the time, the principles

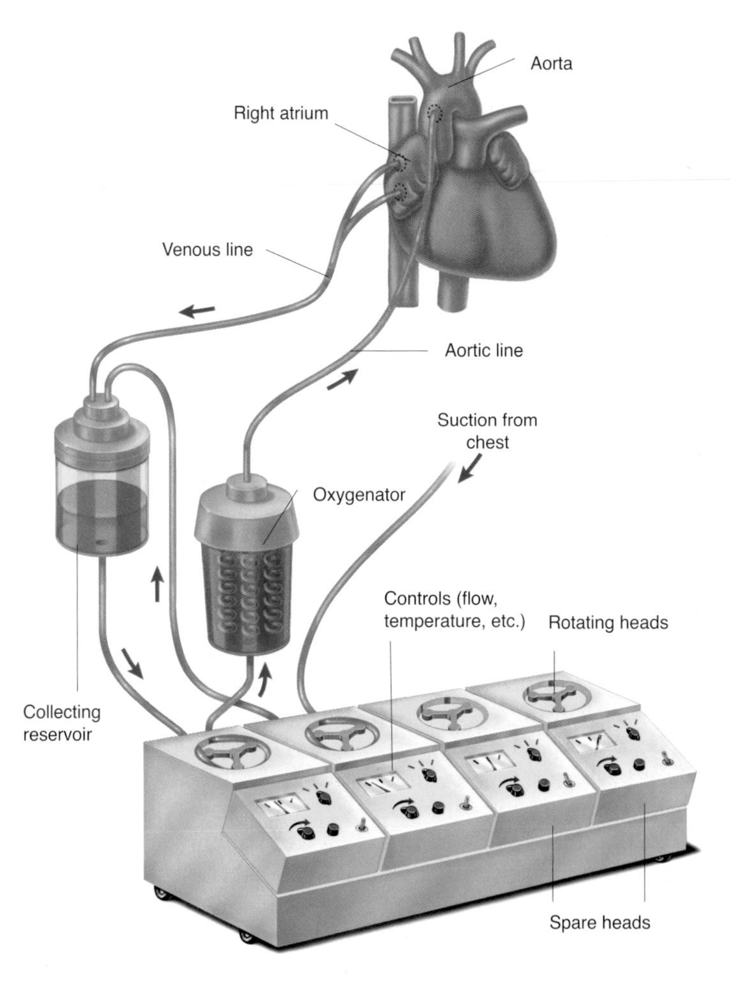

Cardiopulmonary bypass machine.

involved are the same now as they were then.

Although it has been an incredible breakthrough for heart surgery, the basic principles behind it are quite simple. The heart pumps blood to the body and the lungs, so if you are going to stop the heart and lungs, what do you need to do? The answer is, of course, artificially to do the job of the heart, so you need to have a pump. You also need to make sure that oxygen is put into the blood, because the lungs are stopped, so you need an oxygenator. If you can make a machine to fulfil those requirements, you are well on your way to developing the heart–lung machine.

The machine basically works as follows: the surgeon puts a big pipe (venous line) in the right atrium, which collects all the blood returning to the heart through the vena cava. He or she puts another pipe into the aorta near the heart (aortic line). These two pipes are connected by lengths of tubing which pass through the machine.

When the machine is switched on, blood is siphoned down the venous line into the machine where it is oxygenated, and then pumped back into the aortic line. A completely closed circuit then exists, and the heart and lungs can be stopped, because their jobs are being performed artificially. The heart is stopped either electrically or chemically, as we shall explain later, and the lungs are stopped by getting the anaesthetist to switch off the ventilator. Oxygen-rich blood is being circulated around the body to all the organs as required for normal function.

The cardiopulmonary bypass machine is operated by a highly trained specialist called a perfusionist. It is the perfusionist's job carefully to control the machine during the period of cardiopulmonary bypass, when the heart and lungs are switched off. The perfusionist can control several things, such as the rate of flow of the pump, and the temperature of blood passing through. Temperature is important, because the metabolic rate of the body is much lower when cold, and this helps to protect the heart during the time it is not beating, because it requires fewer nutrients and expends less energy.

Traditionally, most heart surgery has been performed at lower temperatures than normal body temperature, commonly between 28°C and 34°C, depending on the preference of the individual surgeon. Much research has been directed at 'warm heart surgery' over the last few years, because it was thought to confer advantages of its own compared with the advantages of cooling as outlined above. It has been scientifically shown that certain forms of warm heart surgery are safe, and for this reason it is becoming more and more widely used. Whichever temperature method is used is safe, however, and makes little difference to the rest of the operation.

Protecting the heart

Unfortunately, when a heart is stopped, its cells will start to get damaged unless there is some way of protecting them. Low temperatures are one way, but this alone is not enough.

The concept of 'myocardial protection' has therefore been developed to deal with this problem, and nearly all heart operations use this. By stopping the heart in a certain way, its energy expenditure and requirements are reduced, and the minimum amount of harm is caused, effectively protecting the heart muscle. There are two broad ways of stopping the heart during cardiopulmonary bypass – one is chemical and one electrical:

- The chemical method involves infusing a solution called cardioplegia directly into the heart. This solution can be either blood or a clear fluid, can be warm or cold, and contains large amounts of potassium. The cardioplegia is forced down the coronary arteries so that it gets to bathe every cell in the heart. The potassium causes the heart to stop beating for a short period of time (up to about half an hour), during which the surgery can take place. The heart starts beating spontaneously once this has worn off, and if the operation has not quite finished, some more cardioplegia can be given to keep the heart still. The advantage of cardioplegia is that it can be topped up as many times as required, which is very useful in particularly long or tricky operations. It is usual to give a repeat or top-up dose every 20 to 30 minutes to keep the heart fully still and protected.

- The electrical method is called intermittent fibrillation, and involves connecting two leads from a machine (called a fibrillator) directly to the heart. When the fibrillator is switched on, the heart stops beating and develops a very fine tremor. The heart can be defibrillated back to beating again with a different machine called a defibrillator. This is done between each bypass graft, to give the heart a rest from the tremor, explaining why the technique is called intermittent.

It does not matter which method is used because they both work very well. Although individual surgeons have their own preferred method, research has not yet clearly demonstrated a great advantage of any one method over another. Most surgeons use the method with which they are most comfortable, but retain the ability to use an alternative technique should the need arise.

An increasing number of operations are now being performed on the beating heart without the need for cardiopulmonary bypass. This is known as off-pump coronary artery bypass or OPCAB and is dealt with later (see page 83).

POSSIBLE COMPLICATIONS

There are a number of potential complications that may occur during cardiac surgery, but fortunately they don't arise very often. As technology and knowledge advance, these operations get safer and safer all the time. Each individual operation has its own particular problems, but many of these are anticipated, and allowed for when calculating individual risks. There are some complications that can occur with any cardiac procedure (see box).

Many of these problems can be attributed to the period of time spent on the heart–lung machine. Although it is a wonderful invention, without which cardiac surgery would barely exist, it is not a normal physiological environment for the body, and some organs may suffer from it.

WHAT MIGHT GO WRONG

- Problems coming off the heart–lung machine
- Bleeding
- Stroke
- Kidney failure
- Breathing difficulties
- Wound infections

Problems coming off the heart–lung machine

The machine takes over the function of your heart and lungs for a variable period of time, while you have your surgery. When the surgery is finished, the heart and lungs need to be started up again, so that the mechanical support can be withdrawn. Usually this is not a problem, but if the heart is quite poorly, it may not be able to start up strongly enough straight away. If this is the case, there are two ways in which the heart can be given some support. The first is with strong, specialised drugs, and the second is with mechanical devices. The most common of these devices is called an intra-aortic balloon pump (balloon pump for short). Less commonly used are ventricular assist devices (VADs).

The drugs that are usually used either increase the force with which the heart muscle contracts, or increase the blood pressure. The balloon pump sits inside the aorta, and eases the work that the heart has to do to create an adequate blood pressure as well as improving the blood flow down the coronary arteries.

If you return to the ICU with either of these means of support, the plan is to ease down their influence gradually over the next few days while the heart recovers, until they can be taken away completely.

Bleeding

There are two main reasons for bleeding excessively after your operation. One is that the components of the blood that cause it to clot are not working properly. This can be fixed by giving these components artificially through drips.

The second is that there is bleeding from small blood vessels that have been cut during the operation, but which have remained hidden when the surgeon was finishing the operation. The only solution to this is for you to go back to theatre so the surgeon can stop these vessels bleeding. This problem

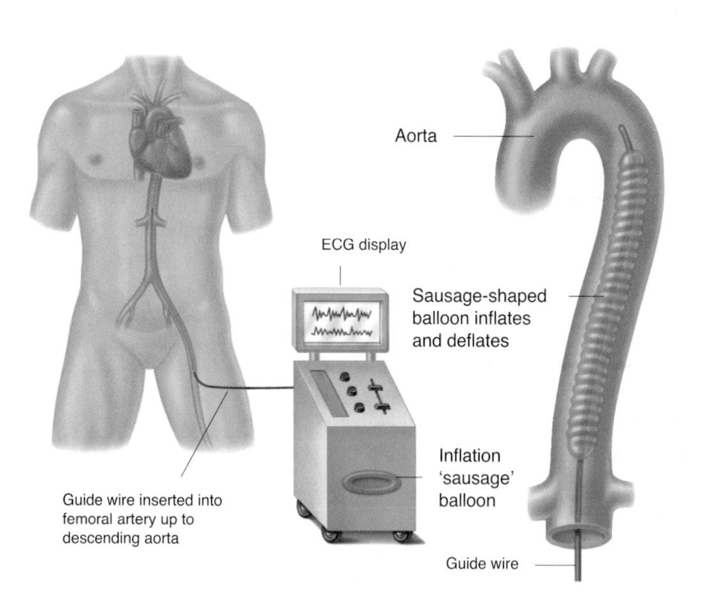

Balloon pump.

affects between two and five patients in every 100. An important part of all heart operations is to leave one or more drains in the chest cavity at the end of the operation. This allows blood to escape so it does not build up and put pressure on the heart, and allows accurate measurement of blood loss. These drains come out of small holes just below your chest scar.

Stroke

A small number of patients have a stroke while they are having their operation. This means that the blood supply to a part of the brain has been interrupted, either because a blood vessel has become blocked by a clot or because a blood vessel bursts and causes bleeding into the surrounding tissue.

Other patients may suffer from a stroke resulting from the presence of severe atherosclerotic disease (furring up) of the main blood vessels that supply the brain. Patients who are known to have this disease usually have an ultrasound of these blood vessels in their neck to see whether anything needs to be done before their heart surgery. It is very difficult to predict who may be affected in this way, so everybody is warned. It may be a small stroke from which the person completely recovers, or it may be a severe one. How serious the outcome is depends on the amount and exact location of the damage.

It is not uncommon for a patient to be slow to wake up after heart surgery, or to be violent and confused. This results partly from the effects of the heart–lung machine and partly from the effects of the anaesthetic. This is not the same as a stroke, and a full recovery is normally reached after a few days. Nevertheless, it can be quite disturbing for the relatives, and reassurances from the doctors and nurses are often required.

A severe stroke may result in paralysis down one side of the face or body. This may be permanent, or the person may recover to a degree, with the help of physiotherapy.

Kidney failure

A small number of people will experience this problem after their operation, but it is usually slightly easier to predict the individuals who face an increased risk than it is with strokes. People with poor kidney function before the operation are more likely to have this failure, and once again this is probably related to time on the heart–lung machine. If you develop kidney failure after the operation, you may have to spend a few days on a kidney machine until they start working again.

Breathing difficulties

This is a much more common

problem, and usually occurs once you have come off the ventilator and started breathing for yourself again. Lying down for a long period of time, as you do when you have an operation, and staying in bed afterwards, causes sputum to build up in your lungs.

As a result some areas of the lungs may collapse. This is particularly likely in smokers, especially those who have smoked right up until their operation. For this reason it is extremely dangerous to smoke in the couple of days before surgery. Chest infections are treated by vigorous physiotherapy, and antibiotics if an infection develops. Sometimes, however, if things do not improve, you may need to go back on the ventilator for a short period of time.

Wound infections

Unfortunately, these are not as rare as they might be and every possible precaution is taken to avoid them. Minor ones tend to heal on their own if treated with antibiotics and meticulous wound care. Major ones can be a real problem, and may even prevent the breastbone from healing. In this case, one or more extra operations are required to clean the infected tissue away and re-close the wound. Overweight people, people with diabetes, people with breathing problems and people on steroids are more likely to develop complications of wound healing.

There is a relatively new technique now available for treating deep-seated infections in both chest and leg wounds. It involves a specialised sponge being inserted into the wound (often in the operating theatre), which is then connected to a powerful suction machine. This machine is often small and portable, allowing ease of movement around the ward. The sponge usually needs to be changed every three days until the infection has settled, after which time the wound can be closed. Sponge treatment of deep wounds is much more comfortable for the patient and has revolutionised the treatment of such conditions.

KEY POINTS

- ✓ Your heart and lungs are stopped for a while during the operation, and you go on to a heart–lung machine
- ✓ Most complications are reversible

Surgery for ischaemic heart disease

CORONARY ARTERY BYPASS GRAFTING

Usually abbreviated to CABG, this is the definitive surgical treatment for ischaemic heart disease (IHD). The concept is simple: you have a blockage or narrowing in a coronary artery, and it is important that blood gets to the area of the heart on the far side of the blockage.

You therefore need to divert the blood flow past the blockage. This can be done by connecting a new tube or conduit to the blood supply on the normal side of the blockage, and connecting the other end to the coronary artery beyond the blockage.

The CABG operation will allow blood to 'bypass' the blockages or narrowings in your coronary arteries. The number of bypasses you have depends upon the number of arteries that are blocked, and the operation is basically the same for each blockage.

So, when people talk about a 'triple bypass' it means that three arteries are blocked, but it is quite common to have a single, double, quadruple or even more bypasses in your operation. The number is not especially important, as long as all arteries with significant narrowing or blockages get bypassed.

In this way a normal blood supply is re-established to all the deprived areas of heart. It is a bit like plumbing, really.

There are several ways of doing this, but they all follow the same broad principles:

- Most operations are performed with the aid of cardiopulmonary bypass (CPB), so that the heart can be stopped to make the surgery easier. There are, however, well-established techniques and equipment to allow CABG to be performed without CPB. There has been extensive development of specialised equipment for stabilisation of the parts of the beating heart to be operated upon, and to keep the

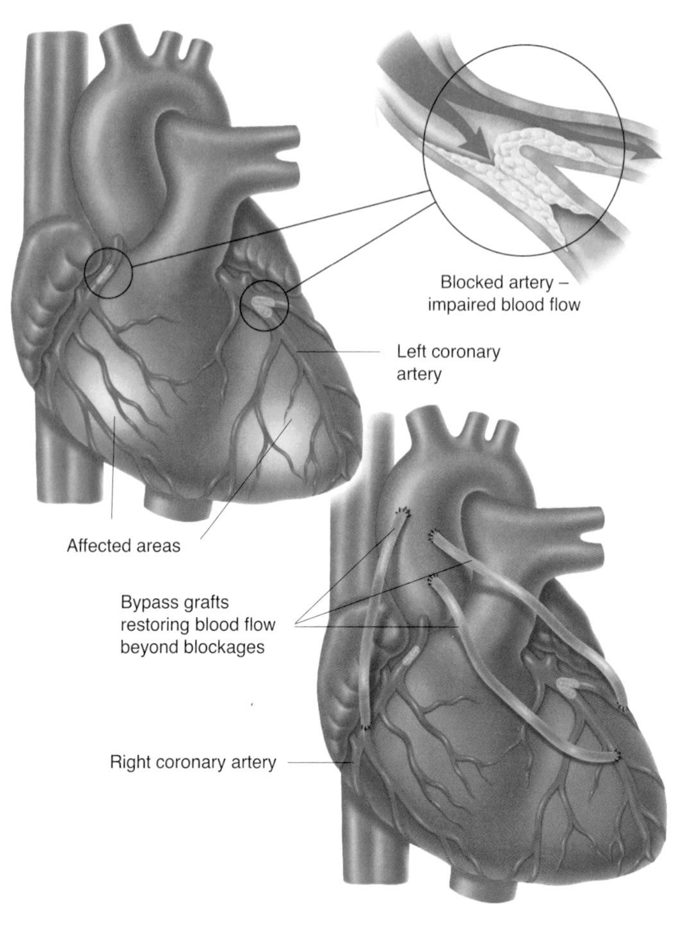

Coronary artery bypass grafts.

operative field clear of blood. This 'off-pump' surgery is becoming more and more popular and has the advantage of avoiding the complications associated with being on the CPB machine. However, these complications are rare anyway, so it is still up to the preference of the individual surgeon as to which technique he or she will use. In general, 'off-pump' surgery is reserved for cases requiring fewer numbers of bypass grafts, although some surgeons will happily use it for almost all cases.

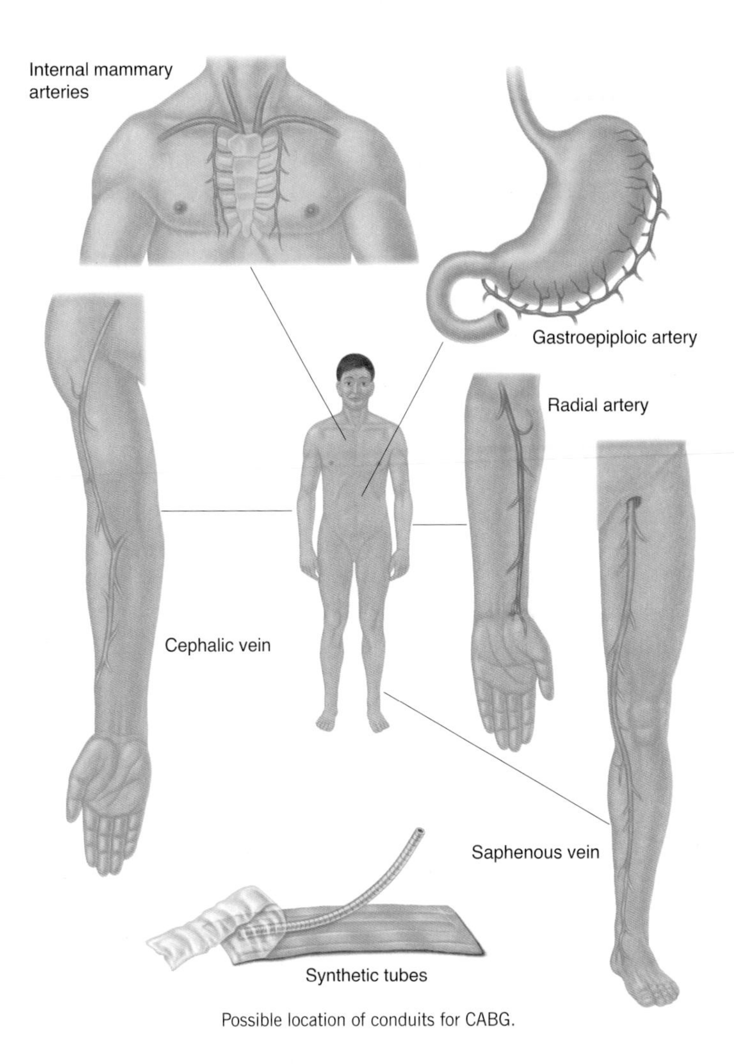

Possible location of conduits for CABG.

- Myocardial protection is needed (see page 41), and the surgeon chooses which method he or she prefers.
- A conduit is needed to connect the vessel before the blockage with the vessel beyond.

Conduits

There are a number of different conduits that can be used, and they are broadly divided into vein, artery and synthetic.

Veins or arteries from your own body are by far the best things to

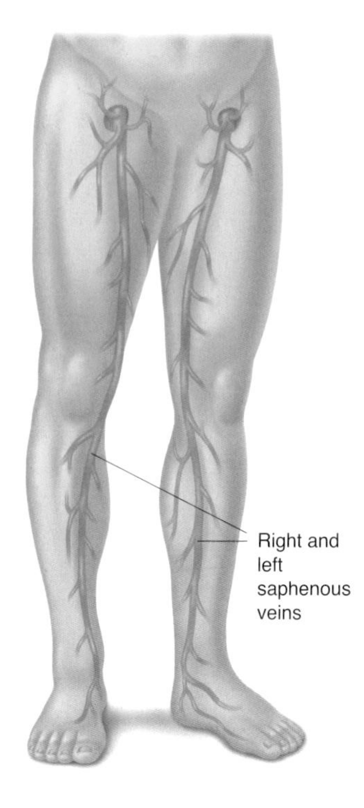

Location of long saphenous veins.

use, because there is no danger of rejection or infection. Not long ago, vein was used in nearly all surgery for CABG, but nowadays arteries are playing a much more dominant role. They are thought by many to be a far superior conduit to vein and there are some surgeons who use only arterial grafts. There is still no conclusive evidence for this, however, and both are excellent options. In fact, the recent innovation in the development of statins, the drugs that keep cholesterol low, is very likely to be a factor in keeping vein grafts open for longer and longer.

- **Vein:** In over 90 per cent of all CABG operations performed, the patient's leg is opened to take out some vein. This is usually the long saphenous vein, a superficial vein on the inside of your leg that runs from your ankle to your groin. This vein is not important to you, and you do not suffer any ill-effects from its removal. It is, in fact, the vein that becomes unsightly when you have 'varicose veins' and is often removed anyway. The amount that is taken out depends on the number of bypasses you need, approximately eight inches being required for each. Other veins from the arm are sometimes used, but only if it is not possible to use the long saphenous vein (for example, if it has been removed for varicose veins, or it is too small). You must be aware, however, that when you wake up, you may have scars on either or both legs, and maybe even your arm, because if the surgeons cannot find any usable vein at first they will move on to the next best place.

- **Artery:** The advantage of using arteries is that blood is already being actively pumped down them. If you can find a relatively unimportant one near the heart, it is only necessary to connect the one end to the coronary artery beyond its blockage, and you have provided a new blood supply to the region. The internal mammary arteries (IMA) are ideally suited for this, and have had a revolutionary effect on CABG surgery. They are located behind the breastbone (sternum), and there are two of them: a left (LIMA) and a right (RIMA). They help in supplying blood to the breastbone, but because this bone has other sources of blood, one or both of them can be disconnected from it.

The LIMA is used in more than 90 per cent of CABG operations. For a 'triple bypass', the most popular choice of surgeons is either the LIMA and two lengths of long saphenous vein (LSV), or the LIMA, the radial artery and one length of LSV. Use of the RIMA is becoming increasingly popular, and some surgeons use it as well as the LIMA for nearly all cases. After the chest has been opened, the surgeon carefully teases away the IMA from the back of the breast-bone, leaving one end connected to the big artery coming from the aorta, and disconnecting the other end from the bone. When disconnected, blood will squirt from the end indicating that it is good enough to use. A temporary clip can be put across the end to prevent it bleeding, and the IMA is now ready to be connected to the coronary artery.

As we have mentioned earlier, arteries are thought by many to be

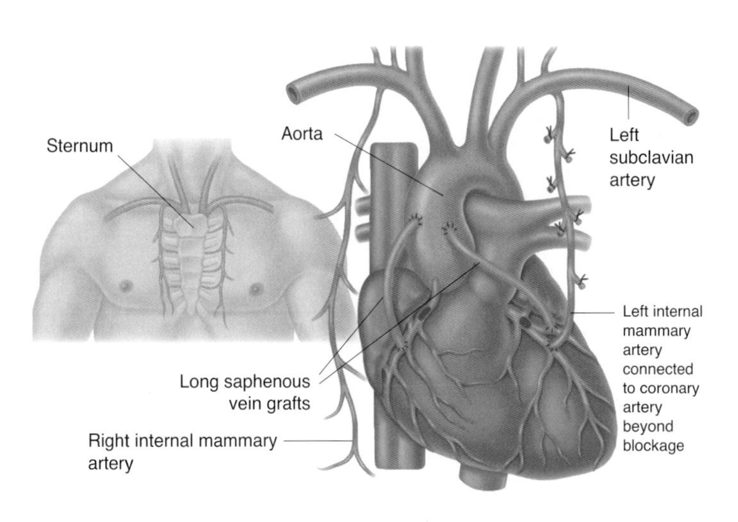

Utilising LIMA for CABG.

better conduits, although there is no substantive proof and there are many trials under way at present in an attempt to prove the benefit. There are some surgeons who are very much in favour of 'total arterial revascularisation' (TAR). This means using arterial conduits, and not veins, for all of the bypasses. This can be done by using both IMAs, combined with either the gastroepiploic artery from the stomach, or the radial artery from the wrist. The gastroepiploic artery is useful because, like the IMA, it lies close to the heart, and only one end

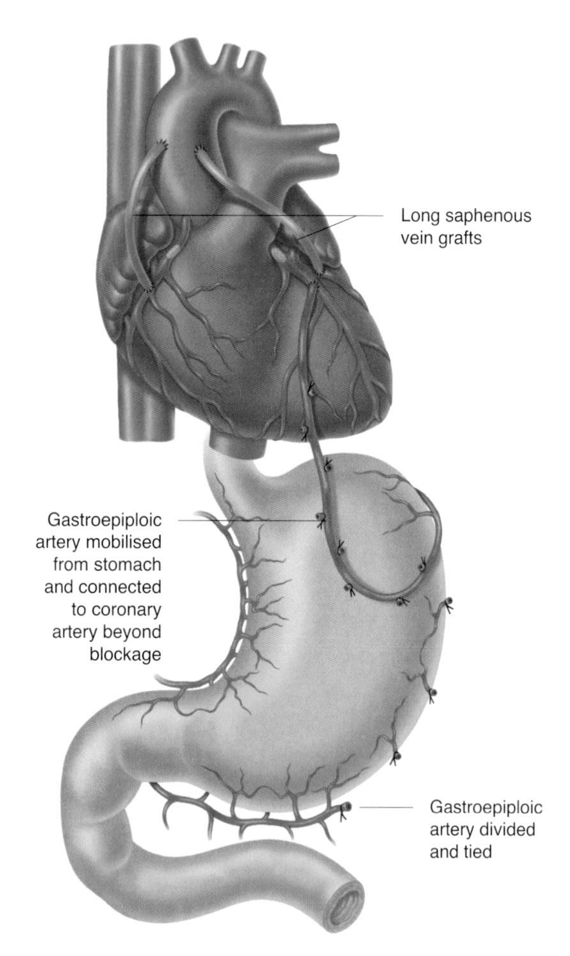

Utilising gastroepiploic artery for CABG.

needs to be disconnected. The disadvantage is that it is in your abdomen, which means a longer operation. The radial artery is in your wrist, and is obviously too far from your heart to be used similarly. In this case it is taken out completely, and used as a 'free graft' where each end is connected to either side of the coronary artery blockage, in much the same way as vein.

- **Synthetic grafts:** These are really a last resort, and are very, very rarely used. They last for a much shorter period of time than any of the other conduits, and are only used if no usable vein or artery can be found in your body. They are usually made of Dacron or Teflon and, although well sterilised, pose a much greater risk of becoming infected, as do any other foreign materials being implanted into your body.

How the operation is done

Your chest is opened down the middle from the 'notch' between your collarbones to the 'V' of your ribcage. Your breastbone is also cut neatly down the middle using a special saw. Once this has been done, it is possible to open your chest cavity surprisingly wide, to get a very good view of the heart. One or both IMAs are then taken down. While this is going on in the

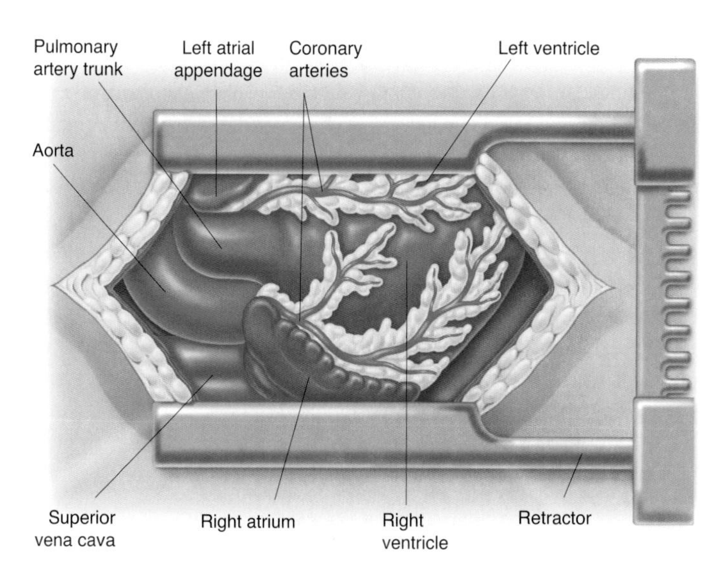

Surgeon's view of open chest cavity.

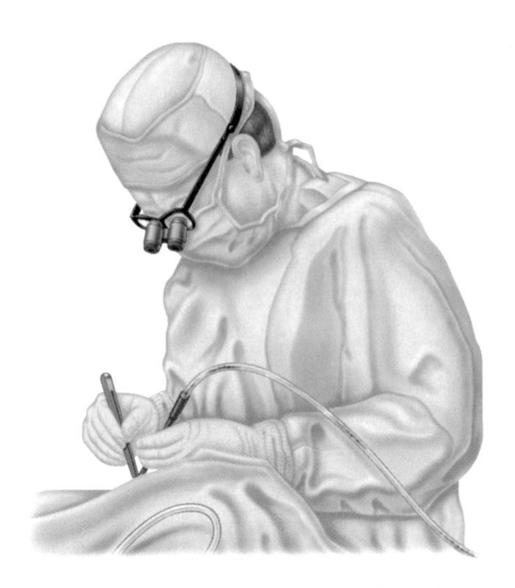

Surgeon using magnifying spectacles (loupes).

chest, a second surgeon is usually taking the vein out of the leg, and if needed a third surgeon can take the radial artery out of the arm (usually the left). When the surgeon at the chest has taken the IMA, the next stage is to put the cardiopulmonary bypass pipes into the aorta and right atrium (see 'Cardiopulmonary bypass', page 38) and connect them to the heart–lung machine. When the surgeon is happy that there is enough conduit, he or she can tell the perfusionist to start the heart–lung machine, and the patient is then 'on bypass' and the CABG can be performed.

The precise order of events depends on the method of myocardial protection used, but the end result is the same. The conduit (vein or artery) is sewn on to the coronary artery beyond the blockage using a very fine stitch, for which the surgeon often uses special magnifying spectacles called loupes. The other end of the conduit is sewn on to the aorta, to a small hole that has been cut in it. In this way, blood pumped up the aorta will pass down the new vein graft to the area of heart beyond the blockage.

An important point to note is that the vein must be sewn in upside-down, because it contains valves and only allows blood to flow in one direction. The free end of the IMA or other arterial grafts is sewn to the coronary artery in a similar way to that described for the vein. The stitches are close enough together to prevent leakage, and after a period of time the join heals just like stitches in your skin.

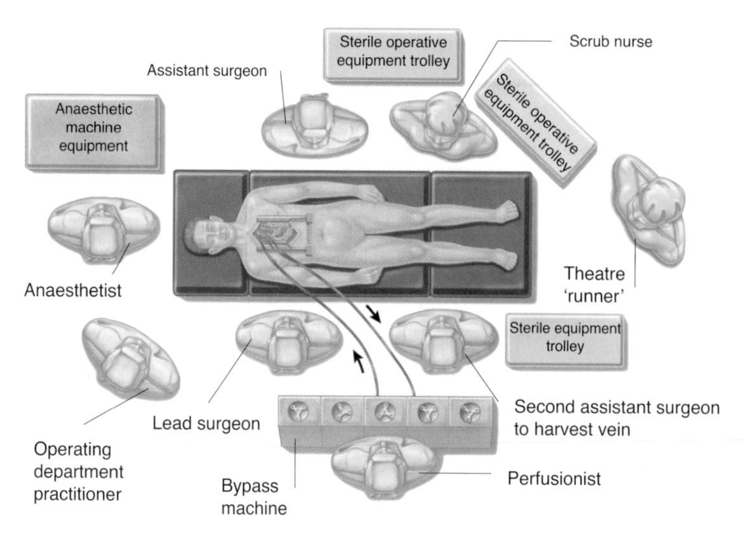

Operation in progress (seen from above).

When the grafts have all been sewn on, it is time to come 'off bypass'. As the operation is performed at a lower temperature for myocardial protection, the perfusionist is asked to warm the patient up before this can happen. After the patient is off bypass, the pipes can be removed, and the chest closed. The breastbone is put together using six to eight stainless steel wires, before the other tissues and skin are sewn up. These wires hold the breastbone together tightly and, within about three to six months, the bone will have healed up itself. The wires, however, remain in place long term. After your operation you will be taken to the ICU.

CABG generally lasts a good period of time, usually in excess of 10 years and often a lot longer. Factors that will keep the bypass grafts 'open' and healthy include good control of diabetes, cholesterol and blood pressure and non-smoking. Failure to control any of these may result in much earlier 'furring up' and blockage of the grafts, with the consequence of heart attack or the need for a repeat operation. If the grafts do not last, your symptoms may start to reappear. This results from the unavoidable fact that the disease process that 'furred' your coronary arteries up in the first place does not go away, and is doing the same to your new conduits. When this happens, you may need to have the operation again, and this is known as a 're-do'. It is similar to the first operation, but technically much more difficult, because the anatomy has been distorted. Finding suitable conduit can be quite tricky too. This is because the best conduit (LIMA and veins) has usually been taken out for the first operation. For all these reasons, your operative risk is proportionally higher.

OTHER SURGICAL PROCEDURES

There are a few other surgical procedures that are performed for IHD, but they are much less common than CABG.

- **Aneurysmectomy:** This means the cutting out and repair of an 'aneurysm' which is a swelling in a dead area of heart muscle caused by a heart attack. If an aneurysm exists, it needs to be inspected carefully during the operation, because if it is thin, it is in danger of rupturing and needs to be repaired. This is a relatively quick and easy procedure.

- **A ventricular septal defect (VSD) repair:** This can be a life-threatening problem and usually means that the person must have emergency surgery. It is a hole that forms in the dividing wall (septum) between the left and right ventricles. The hole is a rupture in a dead piece of muscle, caused by a heart attack. It is relatively rare, but if it does occur, the patient is extremely unwell and the risks are very high.

- **Transmyocardial revascularisation (TMR):** This is an experimental technique that was developed several years ago and initially held a lot of promise. It was thought to be an option for the treatment of patients with severe IHD, but who were not suitable for conventional CABG as a result of very small coronary arteries. It involves the use of a laser to drill about 30 holes in the ventricles of the heart. This is supposed to stimulate the formation of new blood vessels in the substance of the muscle, and therefore relieve the ischaemia. Unfortunately, results have not lived up to expectations and the technique has been largely abandoned. It is still under scrutiny, however, and only appropriate for a small proportion of patients at present, usually those with poor ventricular function and small coronary arteries.

There are very limited positive research data on this technique to date, and it is regarded with a great degree of scepticism by many. For this reason, it has largely been abandoned by most surgeons.

KEY POINTS

- ✓ CABG is the main operation for IHD
- ✓ CABG requires conduits (arteries or veins)

Surgery for valvular heart disease

How the operation is done

The actual opening of the chest, exposure of the heart and insertion of the bypass pipes are effectively the same as for CABG. Cardio-pulmonary bypass and myocardial protection are needed, but conduits are not (unless you are having a combined valve and CABG operation, of course). Once the patient is 'on bypass', and myocardial protection instituted, the specific valve replacement part of the operation can be performed. Before the operation is even started, however, a very important decision needs to be made, and that is choosing which valve to put in.

Choice of valve

There is quite a wide range of artificial heart valves on the market, broadly divided into two categories:

1. Mechanical valves
2. Tissue valves (xenografts).

Within each of these categories there are several different designs. Within the mechanical valve subgroup, the most common types of valves found use single or double tilting discs (mono-leaflet and bi-leaflet, respectively). The 'ball and cage' design which was originally the most popular has been largely superseded by these 'bi-leaflet' valves. Tissue valves may be preserved whole valves from an animal (usually a pig), or may be constructed from the pericardium (the membrane surrounding the heart) of an animal (usually a cow).

The feature that all valves share is that they allow the passage of fluid only in one direction, and prevent it from going the other way. The choice of which valve to use is a combined decision between the surgeon and the patient, because there are many different factors to be considered, and each patient is different and has individual needs.

Broadly speaking, mechanical valves probably last at least 15 to 20 years, but quite often much longer. Tissue valves are a newer invention, and it is not known how long they last, but it is probably a shorter time of around 12 to 15 years. The newest generation of tissue valves may well last even longer than that according to laboratory tests, but unfortunately they haven't been around long enough to measure how long they actually last. When a valve has worn out, a re-do operation is needed to take it out and replace it with yet another new one.

- **Mechanical valves:** These consist of the valve itself mounted within a special ring which is the means by which it is sewn into the heart. The valve component is made of a strong, solid material which has been put through strict testing. The important thing is that it is an artificial material and, like any other artificial material introduced into the bloodstream, is prone to cause clots to develop upon its surface. Clots that form in the bloodstream can be very dangerous, because if they dislodge they can shoot off to distant places such as the brain, causing a stroke. Therefore, if you have a mechanical valve you need to take an anticoagulant drug to thin the blood. This is usually warfarin, and is taken as a small tablet once a day.

If you have a mechanical valve it is important to understand that this commits you to taking warfarin for life. The only difference the warfarin will make to you is that you may bleed a little longer if you cut yourself. This can be a nuisance to some people with physical jobs. It also means that you will need to attend your doctor's surgery or a clinic at regular intervals to check the thinness of the blood. Many people having valve replacements have an irregular heart beat called atrial fibrillation as a result of enlargement of the heart over the years. These people will usually be taking warfarin anyway, and therefore a mechanical valve is probably the best choice. The other potential disadvantage of mechanical valves is that they make a slight clicking noise, and this can be disconcerting to some people. However, most people can hear nothing at all, or perhaps only at times of complete silence.

- **Tissue valves:** These are also called xenografts (*xeno-* comes from the Greek for 'foreign'), and comprise a complete pig's valve, or may be made from pericardium. Whichever of these the valve is made from, they are all mounted in a similar sewing ring to that of mechanical valves. Pigs have similarly sized hearts and valves to humans, and their valves have been

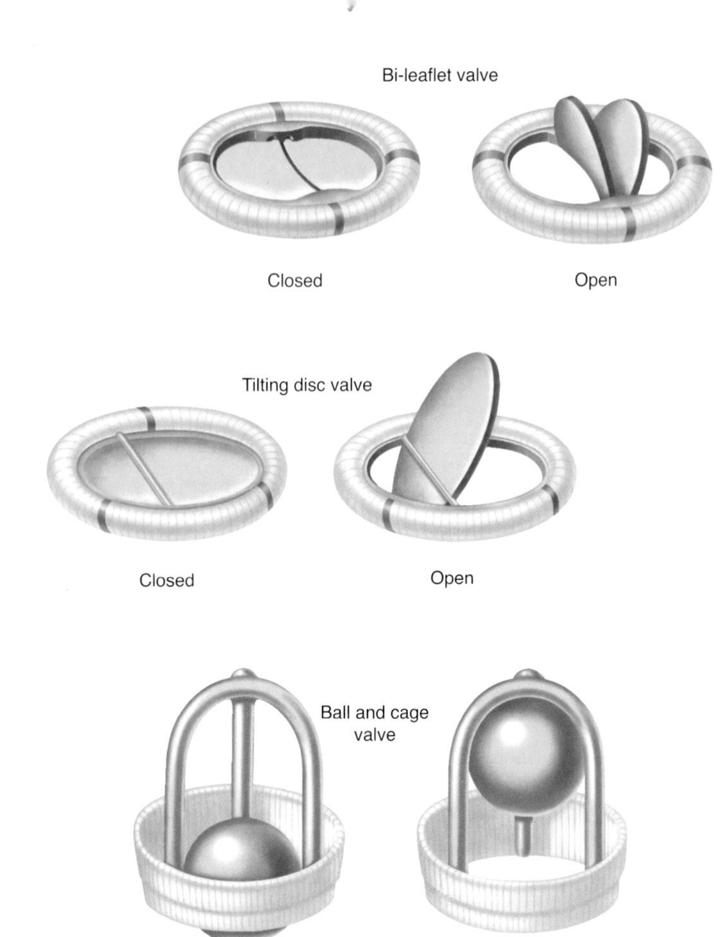

Common types of mechanical valve.

used successfully for many years. All xenografts are specially treated to prevent the body from rejecting them, and to make them stronger. They do not stimulate clot formation, so you don't have to take warfarin for the rest of your life, although you are usually put on it for about six weeks to allow the valve to settle in. Tissue valves are also completely silent.

The choice of valve depends on weighing up the longer durability of a mechanical valve with its disadvantages. In general, if you think your life expectancy is less than 10–15 years, and you will not get as far as a re-do operation, then it may be best to have a xenograft and its lack of disadvantages. Otherwise, it is a decision that is made between you and the surgeon, and is tailored to your individual needs.

Aortic valve replacement

Once the patient is on cardio-pulmonary bypass (CPB), cardioplegia is given to stop the heart, and then the aorta can be opened to gain access to the valve. The old valve is carefully cut out and discarded. The aperture that is left is then measured with an instrument called a 'sizer', because each type of valve comes in a wide range of sizes. The biggest valve that will fit is chosen, and the surgeon then sews the valve ring into place exactly where the old one was removed, and closes the aorta over it. When the perfusionist has warmed the patient up, the heart is restarted and CPB stopped. The pipes can then be removed and the chest is closed as for CABG.

Mitral valve replacement

Mitral valve surgery is technically very similar to aortic valve surgery. The main difference is that the left atrium needs to be opened to expose and cut out the old valve, and there are a number of different approaches to this. The other feature of mitral valve surgery is that, when opening the atrium, there is a chance of disturbing the nerve conduction fibres from the natural pacemaker. This may cause

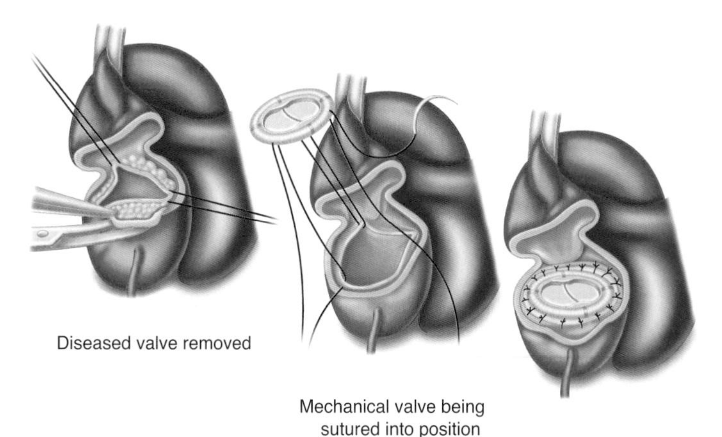

Aortic valve replacement.

rhythm problems when coming 'off bypass' or after the operation, so to guard against this the surgeon attaches some temporary 'pacing wires' to the heart. These come out of your skin just below the chest scar, and can be connected to a pacemaker at any time if required. Usually, they are not needed, and simply (and painlessly) pulled out by a nurse on the ward before you go home. It is not uncommon for temporary pacing wires to be needed in any of the other forms of heart surgery, and some surgeons attach them to nearly all patients. The important thing to realise is that they are not usually needed for more than a day or two, if at all, and they are simply a precaution while the heart recovers from the operation.

Valve repair

A technique that is becoming increasingly popular is valve repair and this is far more common in the mitral valve. Aortic valve repair is still very rare, mainly as a result of the nature of the disease process that causes aortic stenosis (narrowing). Mitral valve repair should always be considered in cases of mitral regurgitation, and is very often possible, depending on the experience of the surgeon. In these cases, a variety of repair techniques is used, including reattaching the cords to the leaflets, cutting out excessive floppy valve tissue, and reducing the overall size of the valve using a special ring. The ultimate aim is to reconstruct a functional valve, which is then tested during the operation. If it is not functional, and the repair has not worked, then it is still possible to replace the valve as above. For valve repair, you still need to undergo a similar operation to replacement and go on the heart–lung machine, but your own valve is repaired rather than replaced. This has obvious advantages, because it means that you preserve your own tissues, and do not have foreign materials implanted in your body.

Other valve surgery

The pulmonary and tricuspid valves are much less frequently operated on than the aortic and mitral ones, but the operative principles outlined above are the same.

There are other operations on your aortic valve, where the whole section of your aorta containing the valve is cut out and replaced with a synthetic tube containing a mechanical valve or sometimes a whole section of animal or human aorta containing the natural valve. These are quite complex operations and involve some different principles to the ones we have discussed.

KEY POINTS

- ✓ Replacement valves may be mechanical or tissue
- ✓ Mechanical valves may last longer but require you to take warfarin for life

Transplantation

Heart transplantation is a last resort for patients whose heart disease is no longer responding to drug therapy, and where there are no other operations or forms of treatment available. They fall into a category that is known as 'end-stage heart failure' and usually have a predicted life expectancy of less than a year. There are many causes for end-stage heart failure, but they all result in the heart's inability to act efficiently as a pump.

Receiving a heart transplant is an enormous undertaking, and only some patients with end-stage heart failure are suitable, on both medical and physical grounds. It is well known that there is a great shortage of donor organs, so they are a very valuable commodity and must not be wasted. For this reason, anyone who is a potential recipient of a heart transplant must be thoroughly assessed at the transplant hospital to see whether they are suitable to go on the waiting list.

If you are referred for an assessment, you will be admitted to the transplant hospital for about three days, and go through a lot of tests and be seen by several doctors and other medical staff. At the end of your assessment, the transplant surgeon will look at all the test results and come and see you to discuss the findings. Some patients are thought to be 'too well' for transplantation, and others 'too unwell'. If you are neither of these you will be put on the waiting list and be given a bleeper which will go off if a heart of the right size and blood group becomes available.

The actual operation can be long and often takes place in the middle of the night. This is because the potential donor needs to have 'brain-stem death' tests performed, and discussions with the relatives need to take place. This all tends to happen during the day and, by the time the transplantation can start, it is usually evening. It can be technically difficult if you have had previous heart surgery, and the normal anatomy has been destroyed. At the end of the operation you go to the ICU, and when everything is stable and your breathing tube has been removed you can be moved back to the ward. You are usually in the ICU a little longer than for other heart operations, because of the extra complications of the procedure and the longer period under anaesthetic.

Once you have had a heart transplant, you will find that your quality of life dramatically changes, and you can do things you never dreamed you would be able to do again. You must take a large number of tablets for life, however. The most important of these are the immunosuppressants that stop you from rejecting your new heart. You will have to take two or three different types of immunosuppressants every day for the rest of your life, but it is worth it because they are very effective. More than 80 per cent of all patients who have a heart transplant live longer than five years, and sometimes much longer.

KEY POINTS

- ✓ There is a drastic shortage of donor organs
- ✓ You will need to take immunosuppressive drugs for life to prevent rejection

Children and heart surgery

There is a whole range of diseases affecting children and young adults that need surgical correction. About eight babies in a thousand are affected by some form of congenital heart disease. It is beyond the scope of this book to cover them all, but some of the basic principles can be laid out. The first important thing to realise is that most of these operations are performed by surgeons who specialise exclusively in this type of surgery. It is a completely different field of expertise to adult cardiac surgery, and is normally carried out in designated children's hospitals with specialised ICU staff and facilities.

Congenital heart disease can range from the straightforward, such as 'hole in the heart', to extremely complicated, where parts of the heart are missing or in the wrong place. The 'hole in the heart' is usually the name given to a condition called atrial septal defect (ASD). This is a hole between the left atrium and the right atrium, allowing blood to pass from one side to the other. As the two sides of the heart are separate circuits, with the right carrying oxygen-poor blood and the left carrying oxygen-rich blood, the mixing can cause problems. Symptoms are worse the bigger the hole is, and this dictates when the operation should be performed, but it is not usually an emergency. Some people only develop problems later on in their lives, particularly during the childhood and adolescent growth spurts, and others have no symptoms at all for their whole life. The straightforward cases can usually be fixed by one simple operation, in which the surgeon sews up or puts a patch over the hole, and there should be no further problems. However, the complicated ones frequently need a whole series of operations over the course of their childhood, and sometimes into adulthood. This is very distressing for both the child and the family, and a lot of support and understanding is needed.

KEY POINTS

- ✓ Children have a completely different range of heart conditions
- ✓ Congenital heart problems may require a series of operations to correct

Surgery for rhythm disturbances

Pacemaker insertion

This is not actually performed by a cardiac surgeon in an operating theatre, but by your cardiologist in the angiography laboratory, or a special room called a 'pacing room'. It is carried out under local anaesthetic and usually takes about an hour. It leaves you with a small scar on the left side of your upper chest. You will only need to stay in hospital for one night.

You may need a pacemaker if you have been found to have a slow heart beat causing symptoms such as dizziness, breathlessness, chest pain or collapse (blackout). There are other indications for pacemaker insertion, such as abnormal rhythms causing symptoms, but these are rarer. There are many different types of pacemakers available and, should you require one, your cardiologist will decide which type suits you the best. All pacemakers can be programmed to make the heart beat at a specific rate, and this should relieve your symptoms.

The conduction system may be damaged during some heart operations, particularly those involving the mitral valve. This may require pacemaker insertion as described above before you leave hospital.

Pulmonary vein ablation

One of the most common forms of rhythm disturbance is an irregular heart beat called atrial fibrillation (AF), and it affects hundreds of thousands of people in the UK. One in 100 people aged over 65 suffer from AF, and they need to take special drugs and attend regular clinics. AF can exist in two main ways: established AF, which is present all the time, and paroxysmal AF, which comes and goes from time to time and usually gives symptoms of palpitations.

There are now new surgical treatments for AF that have about a 75 to 80 per cent success rate. This form of treatment is called pulmonary vein ablation (PVA). It is probably not worth going through the whole process of having your chest opened to have one of these procedures, but if you are having heart surgery for another reason and you have AF, your surgeon might recommend that you have this performed at the same time. It only adds about 20 minutes to the operation and involves 'burning' a pattern around the electrical conduction tissue of your heart, using radiofrequency, microwaves or ultrasound. It is very safe and adds minimal risk to your operation with a huge potential benefit if successful.

Even more innovative is the current development of minimally invasive ablation equipment that will allow PVA to be performed without opening the chest, but through 'keyhole surgery' instead. The potential for this is enormous because a huge amount of NHS money is being spent on drugs and hospital treatment for the many people with AF.

KEY POINTS

- ✓ Pacemakers are inserted, under local anaesthetic, by a cardiologist, or heart specialist, not a surgeon
- ✓ Atrial fibrillation affects hundreds of thousands of people in the UK and can be treated by pulmonary vein ablation

After your operation

When you wake up after your operation, you will be in the intensive care unit (ICU). When you are fit enough not to require continuous attention, you can be moved back to the ward. This decision is made by the doctors and nurses on the ICU, and really requires you to be breathing efficiently without help, and not to be on any mechanical or strong drug support.

Sometimes, if you are suitable, and your operation has gone really well, you will be woken up quite quickly and your breathing tube removed (extubated). If all is well, you can then go back to the ward on the same day, rather than spending a night on the ICU. This is known as 'fast-tracking', and is a useful process, because it creates an extra bed on the ICU, which means that another patient can have his or her operation.

Intensive care unit

Some ICUs are specifically for heart surgery patients, and others are 'general' ICUs, which cater for a mixture of patients requiring intensive treatment.

Whichever type you are in, you will be looked after continuously by a specially trained nurse for whom you are the only patient, and by an anaesthetist who is in the ICU at all times. You will always arrive in ICU after your operation connected to the ventilator, and a number of other drips and monitors, depending on your condition (see table on pages 72–3). It should be stressed that all patients arrive back connected to a frightening array of equipment. This is entirely normal and does not necessarily mean that anything is wrong.

As soon as you are settled in and everything is stable, the nurses will try to 'wean' you from the

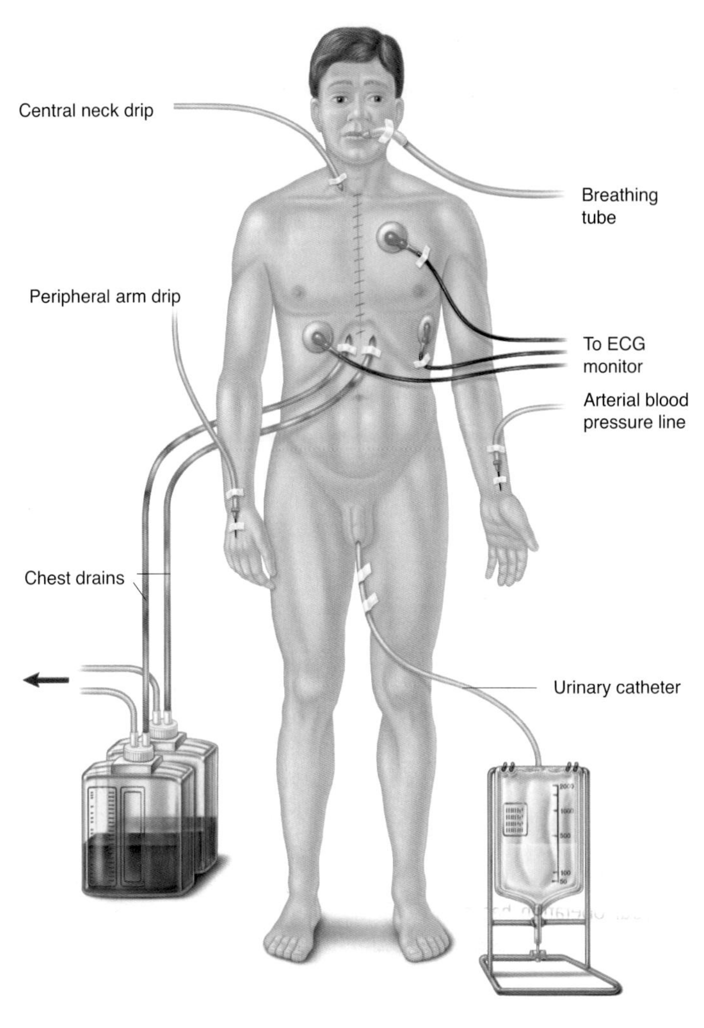

Intensive care unit.

ventilator. In other words, they'll try to wake you up and get you breathing for yourself. They monitor the amount of oxygen in your blood and, when the time is right, will extubate you. This can take place any time from a couple of hours after your operation, to days or weeks later. The ventilator is the only part of the support system that cannot be provided anywhere other than the ICU, so you cannot go back

Routine procedure in ICU	Reason
Breathing tube	To breathe for you, while your paralysed muscles recover from the anaesthetic
Arterial blood pressure line	To monitor your blood pressure continuously
Central neck drip	For giving continuously infused drugs and fluids, and to monitor how much fluid you have in your body
Peripheral arm drip	For 'one-shot' drugs such as antibiotics, and for infusion of fluids
Urinary catheter	To measure how much urine you are producing, which gives an indication of your kidney function, and whether your body has enough fluid inside. This is important because you are asleep so, if you are too dry, you will not be able to complain of thirst
ECG monitor	To observe heart rate, heart rhythm and any abnormalities
Chest drains	There is always a bit of 'oozing' to begin with after heart surgery and, if the blood built up inside the chest, it would compress the heart. The drains let all

	the 'ooze' out, and also alert the staff if there is too much, which would require the chest to be re-opened to stop the bleeding
Sometimes required in ICU	**Reason**
Extra drips for drugs	Some patients require less common drugs to help them recover, and each drug given usually goes through a different drip
Balloon pump	See page 42–3
Kidney machine	Rarely, the kidneys go into failure after heart surgery. The kidneys remove the waste products from the body, which cause harm if not expelled. The kidney machine is a way of doing their job of removing this waste, and is usually only a temporary measure until the kidneys 'wake up' again
Pulmonary artery catheter	This is another drip that is usually inserted into a neck vein, and passed down this into the heart. It is connected to a heart monitor, and can give the doctors a number of important measurements of the heart's function. These special measurements are useful in deciding which supportive drugs to give

to the ward unless you are extubated. All the other drips and devices will gradually be removed over the next two to three days if all is well, but this can take place on the ward.

Ward stay

You will usually go back to the ward the day after your operation. If there have been complications you may stay on the ICU longer, and if you are fast-tracked you may return on the same day. When you arrive back on the ward, you will usually spend the first day or so in a special area called the high dependency unit (HDU). This simply means that the nurses can keep a closer eye on you until all your drips and tubes have been removed. As you get stronger, and continue to improve, you will be moved to the normal part of the ward. Your rehabilitation starts as soon as you reach the ward, and will be dealt with in the next section.

Most people go home about five days after their operation, as soon as the staff (doctors, nurses and physiotherapists) feel that they are capable.

KEY POINTS

- ✓ Everybody goes to ICU after the operation
- ✓ You usually go home after five or six days

Getting back to normal

Your rehabilitation after heart surgery begins immediately and continues for an indefinite period of time. This period of time is very variable, and depends upon your speed of recovery and return to a normal way of life. Each person is different and may have individual problems. Rehabilitation should also consider the needs of your family and friends, and care is taken to keep them informed every step of the way. During the operation itself, your relatives are very welcome to stay in the hospital, but it is normally a better idea to go home, because you are likely to be asleep for at least ten hours in total. They will be informed about any changes, and told of the earliest time to come and visit you. It is understandable that many people may be concerned, and want to come and visit you after your operation. You will be extremely tired after it, and visitors are surprisingly hard work, so it is advisable just to see your immediate family and closest friends for the first few days. The ward staff will notice if you are getting very tired and may ask some visitors to leave. It is important that they do not get upset about this, as it is all in the interests of your recovery.

Immediately after you have been extubated, an oxygen mask will be placed over your nose and mouth. You will be aware of a loud hissing noise that this mask makes. Do not worry about this, because it is only the oxygen being moistened, or 'humidified', before you receive it. You will also receive the attentions of a physiotherapist, who will help you to take deep breaths and practise coughing. If you have been a smoker, you will receive extra attention and 'bullying' from the physiotherapist, because there will almost certainly be a lot of 'muck' on your chest that needs to be brought up.

You may feel very dry, and want a drink. This is fine, but your anaesthetic drugs may make you quite nauseous, so it is advisable to take only sips for the first couple of hours.

You may also find that it hurts to swallow, so be careful. If drinking does make you sick, don't worry, because you will be getting plenty of fluids through your drips, and the nursing staff will give you some anti-sickness drugs.

Pain relief

This is, quite rightly, one of the main concerns of most patients, and the staff will make your comfort a priority. On the ICU, you will automatically be receiving strong painkillers directly into your bloodstream through one of your drips. The dose can be adjusted according to your needs, but may make you feel quite sleepy. You will continue receiving your painkillers in this way, i.e. intravenously, until after your return to the ward and until your pain can be controlled adequately with tablets.

How much painkiller is needed varies enormously between individuals, so take what you need and not what other people tell you that they took. The amount that you need is that which will allow you to achieve all your rehabilitation targets, and this is particularly important after you get home.

Back on the ward

Although it may not seem like it at the time, your return to the ward is a sign of progress. You will probably feel sleepy most of the time to start with; this is a combination of your painkillers and the fact that your operation takes a lot out of you. You will find that, on the second day after your operation, you feel much better, and you will be encouraged to get out of bed and start walking. Initially, the ward staff and physiotherapist will help you, especially getting in and out of bed. Your chest, back and shoulders may feel stiff, and early mobilisation will help to ease much of this stiffness and other aches and pains. You will receive instructions on gentle exercises for your shoulders and arms.

Support stockings

If you have had CABG, involving the removal of vein from your leg(s), you will have to wear special support stockings during this period. These stockings help to reduce swelling of your legs and ankles while the wound heals, and also protect against the formation of dangerous blood clots in your calves (deep venous thrombosis). You should not cross your legs as this encourages clot formation. Wear your stockings during the day for about four weeks after the operation, unless told otherwise by

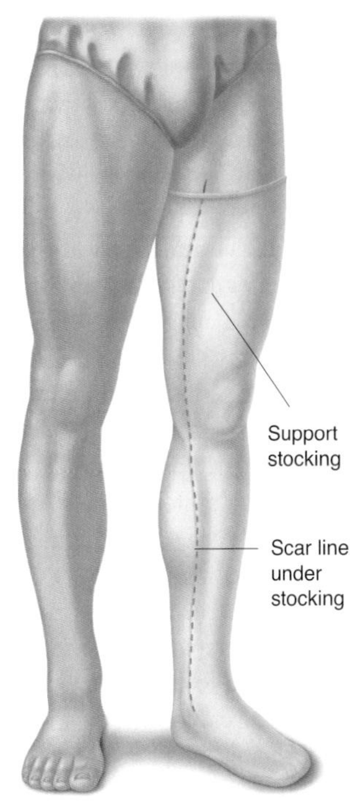

Purpose of support stockings.

your doctor. You should make sure that there are no creases or wrinkles in the stockings because this defeats their purpose. Before you are discharged, you may be given some advice on foot and leg exercises. These are helpful in avoiding stiffness, and should continue for several weeks.

HYGIENE

Once again, just for the first few days, you will need help from the staff for some normal, routine things. As soon as they feel you are ready, you will be able to have a shower or bath under supervision. You may find this surprisingly tiring initially. You might also find that shampooing your hair, brushing your teeth and shaving cause your arms to ache and feel tired. You should not try to rush these tasks early on, and sit down or take a rest if you need to.

Showering is probably easier than bathing, but a stool is useful, particularly to rest and to wash your feet. Try not to have the water too hot, as this may make you feel dizzy or light-headed.

For the first few days, there may be a small amount of blood or fluid discharging from your wounds. This is normal but the ward staff will keep a close eye on their progress, and ensure that they are kept clean, dry and well-dressed. You should also expect some amount of bruising around your wounds. It is quite safe to allow your wounds to get wet, but make sure that they are nice and dry when you have finished washing. The best way to dry your wounds is by 'dabbing' at them, rather than rubbing, and this is also more comfortable.

EATING AND DRINKING

You may notice that your appetite is reduced during the early recovery period, and you may feel nauseous as mentioned earlier. It is probably more important to have adequate amounts to drink during this period, and your fluid intake will be carefully monitored by the ward staff. It is inadvisable to have too many fizzy drinks for the first few days as you may feel 'bloated' anyway. If your bowel habit changes, do not be alarmed. Constipation is common, and results partly from the anaesthetic drugs and painkillers. A gentle laxative tablet is usually all that is required.

Many people benefit from advice on how to eat a healthier diet after heart surgery, because a poor diet may have been one of the factors that contributed to your getting heart disease in the first place. Your GP can give you this advice or refer you to a dietitian and there are plenty of booklets available on healthy eating.

Depression

It is a very common event suddenly to feel quite depressed about four or five days after your operation. This contrasts with the feeling of happiness and euphoria that you may have felt after 'getting through' the surgery. Tears are not uncommon, and you may experience uncharacteristic mood swings. Rest assured, this will not last, and you will be back to normal in a very short time. It sometimes helps to talk to other patients, or staff who have had a lot of experience of this.

Discharge

You and your family will usually be given a couple of days advanced warning about a proposed date for discharge. There is usually a 'pre-discharge' meeting with the nurses and physiotherapists, so that you or your family can ask any questions.

You will usually have some routine blood tests, an ECG and a chest X-ray performed a day or two before you are discharged. Any non-absorbable stitches or pacing wires are also removed the day before you leave. If there are any stitches that must stay, or if your wound is still a little 'oozy', arrangements will be made for a district nurse to come and visit you to take care of this.

In some instances, and for a number of reasons, you may not be ready for home but you are too well for hospital care. In such cases, you may be transferred to a convalescence area for a short while, until you get your strength up. This is carefully arranged for you well in advance, and is usually somewhere close to your home.

It is important to have a relative or friend to look after you to begin with when you do go home. Your GP will get a letter on your discharge, so should be aware that you have had surgery and are back in the community.

Any problems that you may have can initially be referred to your

GP, who can take care of most things. Any specific problems that the GP cannot deal with should be referred back to the team that did your operation. The GP will usually make this referral after seeing you, but if there is a major problem, or you cannot get hold of the GP, remember that there is always somebody in the hospital who can answer your questions over the telephone.

MEDICATIONS

On discharge, you will be given one week's supply of whatever tablets you are taking. You will find that many of the drugs you needed to take before your operation have been stopped, because you don't need them any more. Your GP will receive a letter when you are discharged, and will need to write you a prescription for continuing doses of your drugs.

GOING HOME

In preparation for your journey home, a soft towel or small pillow may reduce seatbelt discomfort. You may feel a bit anxious when you first arrive home after leaving the safe environment of the ward. This feeling isn't at all unusual, and soon disappears. It is a good idea to have a member of the family or a friend at home with you for the first few weeks until you have readjusted.

EXERCISE

Before you go home, you will need to be able to walk unassisted up and down stairs. The physiotherapist will help you with this, and assess your abilities. You may find that short walks of five to ten minutes are best during the first few days. Initially, take walks in familiar environments such as your house and garden.

When you first leave the house, it is best to have company, and to keep the house in sight. As the days progress, you will be able to walk longer distances, and for longer periods of time, even when you are on your own. You shouldn't try walking up hills until you are stronger. You're likely to feel a little short of breath or tired during the early days. You may also feel some discomfort along the shin bone, and in your legs in general.

Your exercise programme will realistically take four to six weeks until you reach a significant level of ability. Your physiotherapist will have given you guidelines and goals before you left hospital, and these will have been tailored to you as an individual. Walking is one of the best forms of rehabilitation at this stage. Try to maintain a good posture, and keep your shoulders down and back. It may help to swing your arms gently or clasp them lightly behind your back. Beware of exercises that may cause the sternum to separate, such as press-ups.

Your physiotherapist will also give you instructions on a range of exercises for your shoulders and arms and it is important to continue these when you are at home. Muscular aches across the shoulders and aching in the upper arms are both common. Gently circling your shoulders, forwards, backwards and upwards, will maintain suppleness. Before you attempt any of your exercise routines, it is a good idea to take your painkillers.

Do not be over-ambitious during the first few days or weeks. You will tire easily, and become frustrated. The most common 'rehabilitation' exercises are walking, swimming and cycling, and many people continue these for life.

Sleeping

Do not be tempted to move your bed downstairs. Your physiotherapist will ensure that you can manage stairs before you leave hospital, so there is no need for this. If you have been taking sleeping tablets in hospital, try to ease yourself off them as soon as you can. You are allowed to sleep in any position you like: find the one that is most comfortable for you. It is up to you whether you share a bed with your partner during the initial period after surgery. Some people prefer a separate bed to maximise uninterrupted sleep. Many patients continue the hospital practice of an afternoon nap, but as your night-time sleep improves, the need for this should decrease.

Your wounds

There will not usually be any problems with the healing of your wounds, but in the event of any of the following, you should contact your GP:

- Persisting redness
- Redness spreading into the surrounding skin
- New or worsening discharge
- New or worsening pain or tenderness.

The top part of your chest wound may remain quite swollen, interfering with buttons or tie knots. This may take several weeks to settle. A numb or 'dead' feeling is also quite common along both your chest wound and your leg wound. This results partly from the unavoidable cutting of some of the tiny skin nerves, but in the case of your chest wound, it is a result of the IMA being taken down from the back of your breastbone. Loose clothing will cause less irritation to these areas until they heal.

Driving

Most surgeons will ask you not to drive for four to six weeks after your operation, usually until you have seen them in clinic. You do not have to inform the DVLA if you have had a routine recovery from a routine operation. If you plan to continue as an LGV or PCV driver, you will need to notify the DVLA. It is a legal requirement to inform your insurance company when your heart condition is diagnosed, and tell them details of operations and complications.

Your sex life

Starting to have sex again after heart surgery can be fraught with unnecessary worry. Sexual intercourse is a form of physical activity, but it will not place a dangerous strain on your heart. You need to discuss this with your partner, because he or she may be equally anxious, but both your fears can be allayed. As with any form of physical activity, do only what you think you can comfortably manage. Familiar and comfortable surroundings help to ease any remaining worries. If you find that you are experiencing problems in resuming sexual activity, you should seek the advice of a health professional recommended by your GP.

Smoking

Smoking after heart surgery is insanity, particularly if you have IHD. The disease process that narrowed your coronary arteries causes narrowings in the new conduits in a much quicker time and, if you smoke, you will accelerate that process hugely. It will also worsen any breathing difficulties and chest infections you may have had in the recovery period.

Returning to work

The timing of your return to work depends upon both you and the type of work. Light non-manual work can be resumed much sooner than heavy manual work. In general, a period of eight to twelve weeks should be set aside for recovery. There will be no problem in getting 'sick certificates' from either your GP or your surgeon.

Clinic appointments

You will see a member of the surgical team in the clinic four to eight weeks after your operation. If you have had CABG, you will then usually be discharged to the care of your GP, but you may also be given an appointment with your cardiologist. If you have had a valve replacement, it is not uncommon to have further follow-up appointments and some surgeons will want to see you every year. Other surgeons, however, are happy to discharge you to the care of your GP or cardiologist. If you have any complications or other problems you can be seen as often as is required, and appointments can be made urgently if needed.

If you have had a mechanical valve replacement, you will also need to attend an anticoagulation clinic to monitor your warfarin therapy. When your warfarin dose is stable, you will only need to attend these clinics every four to six weeks to begin with, then even less frequently as directed by the clinic or your own doctor.

KEY POINTS

- ✓ Your rehabilitation exercises are important
- ✓ After a couple of months you should be back to normal

Recent advances

As with all fields of medicine, research is moving rapidly, and there are always new developments. It would be impossible to cover everything, but we shall deal briefly with some of the most common.

OPCAB

Off-pump coronary artery bypass (OPCAB) surgery is probably the most widely used of the new innovations. A continuously evolving range of new heart stabilisation devices is on the market, allowing safe and effective surgery for appropriate patients. As OPCAB surgery does not require cardiopulmonary bypass, it has the advantages of protection from all the potential bypass-related complications such as stroke. There are a growing number of surgeons who now perform the majority, if not all, of their CABG operations using the OPCAB method. Results of trials to demonstrate a clear advantage over conventional surgery are, however, still awaited. It is not possible to perform valve surgery without cardiopulmonary bypass.

Minimally invasive surgery and robotics

So-called 'keyhole surgery' has been possible for a number of years in some specialities, but is becoming more and more popular in certain areas of heart surgery. It can be performed for CABG, and even valve replacements now, as technology continues to advance. It basically involves a much smaller, or cosmetic, incision, often in the skin fold beneath the left breast, and a couple of small 'stab' incisions which will allow the passage of a telescope or instrument. CABG can sometimes be performed without CPB, but this is technically demanding. This type of surgery is only appropriate for certain patients, but the results are promising. A further development on the minimally invasive techniques available is robotic assisted surgery. The surgeon can perform operations such as CABG and even valve replacement by sitting on the other side of the room in a console, much like a machine at an amusement arcade. He or she then controls computerised instruments, which send instructions to the real instruments that are operating on the patient. This may seem unbelievable, but, although still uncommon, it has been proved to work safely.

Xenotransplantation

This is a very topical subject in research, the results of which are eagerly awaited. It involves breeding pigs which have had their genes modified so as to create hearts that can be transplanted into humans without danger of rejection. The breeding has been taking place for some years now, and the scientists say that they are nearly ready. Unfortunately, human donors currently remain the only source of hearts for people requiring a transplant, and they are extremely scarce. This exciting development would be a major breakthrough if successful.

Artificial hearts

The total artificial heart (TAH) would be another option to xenotransplantation in treating end-stage heart disease. Much research has gone into this, and a successfully implanted long-term human device is still elusive; however, there are some that are getting very close. It has been possible to keep people alive on such devices for increasing periods of time, while they wait for a donor to emerge for routine transplantation, but nothing has been shown to be viable for long-term use.

Something in more common use, but still rare, is the ventricular assist device (VAD), which is used in a similar way to a balloon pump for appropriate patients who have problems coming off the heart–lung machine.

Polymer heart valves

The fact that neither mechanical nor tissue valves are the perfect solution has led scientists to carry out a lot of research combining the best features of each type, and avoiding the disadvantages. Work with polymers has been exciting and several groups have got very close to producing a polymer valve that is ready for human implantation after many years of animal testing. Polymer valves have more strength and durability than tissue valves, therefore lasting longer, but the patient does not need to take warfarin for life as he or she would with mechanical valves.

At present polymer heart valves are in the final stages of testing, but they are likely to be a third alternative in the near future.

KEY POINTS

- ✓ 'Keyhole surgery' is becoming more popular in some areas of heart surgery
- ✓ Future transplants could be of genetically engineered hearts or artificial hearts but these are still in the development stage

Useful addresses

ASH (Action on Smoking and Health)
102–108 Clifton Street
London EC2A 4HW
Tel: 020 7739 5902
Fax: 020 7613 0531
Email: enquiries@ash.org.uk
Website: www.ash.org.uk

National organisation with local branches. Campaigns on anti-smoking policies. Offers free information on website or for sale from headquarters. Catalogue on request.

Benefits Enquiry Line
Tel: 0800 882200
Minicom: 0800 243355
Website: www.dwp.gov.uk
N. Ireland: 0800 220674

Government agency giving information and advice on sickness and disability benefits for people with disabilities and their carers.

British Heart Foundation
14 Fitzhardinge Street
London W1H 6DH
Tel: 020 7935 0185
Fax: 020 7486 5820
Helpline: 08450 708070
Website: www.bhf.org.uk

Funds research, promotes education and raises money to buy equipment to treat heart disease. Information and support available for people with heart conditions. Via Heartstart UK, arranges training in emergency life-saving techniques for lay people.

Chest, Heart and Stroke, Northern Ireland
22 Great Victoria Street
Belfast BT2 7LX
Tel: 028 9032 0184
Fax: 028 9033 3487
Email: mail@nichsa.com
Helpline: 0845 769 7299
Website: www.nichsa.com

Aims to promote the prevention of, and alleviate the suffering resulting from, chest, heart and stroke illnesses in Northern Ireland through advice and information.

Chest, Heart and Stroke, Scotland
65 North Castle Street
Edinburgh EH2 3LT
Tel: 0131 225 6963
Fax: 0131 220 6313
Email: admin@chss.org.uk
Helpline: 0845 077 6000
Website: www.chss.org.uk

Aims to improve the quality of life for people in Scotland affected by chest, heart and stroke illness through medical research, advice and information, and support in the community.

Heart UK
7 North Road
Maidenhead
Berks SL6 1PE
Tel: 01628 628638
Fax: 01628 628698
Email: ask@heartuk.org.uk
Website: www.heartuk.org.uk

Offers information, advice and support to people with coronary heart disease and especially those at high risk of familial hyper-cholesterolaemia. Members receive a bi-monthly magazine.

NHS Smoking Helpline
Tel: 0800 169 0169
Website: www.givingupsmoking.co.uk

For advice, help and encouragement on giving up smoking. Specialist advisers available to offer on-going support to those who genuinely are trying to give up smoking. Can refer to local branches. Pregnancy smoking helpline: 0800 169 9169.

National Institute for Health and Clinical Excellence (NICE)
MidCity Place
71 High Holborn
London WC1V 6NA
Tel: 020 7067 5800
Fax: 020 7067 5801
Email: nice@nice.nhs.uk
Website: www.nice.org.uk

Provides national guidance on the promotion of good health and the prevention and treatment of ill health. Patient information leaflets are available for each piece of guidance issued.

Smoking Quitlines (Quit)
211 Old Street
London EC1V 9NR
Tel: 020 7251 1551
Fax: 020 7251 1661
Helpline: 0800 002200
Email: reception@quit.org.uk
Website: www.quit.org.uk

Offers advice on giving up smoking. Separate helpline for:
Scotland: 0800 848 484 (12 noon–12 midnight)

Stroke Association
Stroke House
240 City Road
London EC1V 2PR
Fax: 020 7490 2686

Helpline: 0845 303 3100
Email: stroke@stroke.org.uk
Website: www.stroke.org.uk

Funds research and provides information; now specialising only in stroke. Local support groups.

THE INTERNET AS A SOURCE OF FURTHER INFORMATION

After reading this book, you may feel that you would like further information on the subject. One source is the internet and there are a great many websites with useful information about medical disorders, related charities and support groups. Some websites, however, have unhelpful and inaccurate information. Many are sponsored by commercial organisations or raise revenue by advertising, but nevertheless aim to provide impartial and trustworthy health information. Others may be reputable but you should be aware that they may be biased in their recommendations. Remember that treatment advertised on international websites may not be available in the UK.

Unless you know the address of the specific website that you want to visit (for example, familydoctor.co.uk), you may find the following guidelines helpful when searching the internet.

There are several different sorts of websites that you can use to look for information, the main ones being search engines, directories and portals.

Search engines and directories

There are many search engines and directories that all use different algorithms (procedures for computation) to return different results when you do a search. Search engines use computer programs called spiders, which crawl the web on a daily basis to search individual pages within a site and then queue them ready for listing in their database.

Directories, however, consider a site as a whole and use the description and information that was provided with the site when it was submitted to the directory to decide whether a site matches the searcher's needs. For both there is little or no selection in terms of quality of information, although engines and directories do try to impose rules about decency and content. Popular search engines in the UK include:

google.co.uk
aol.co.uk
msn.co.uk
lycos.co.uk
hotbot.co.uk
overture.com
ask.co.uk
espotting.com

looksmart.co.uk
alltheweb.com
uk.altavista.com

The two biggest directories are:

yahoo.com
dmoz.org

Portals

Portals are doorways to the internet that provide links to useful sites, news and other services, and may also provide search engine services (such as msn.co.uk). Many portals charge for putting their clients' sites high up in your list of search results. The quality of the websites listed depends on the selection criteria used in compiling the portal, although portals focused on a specific group, such as medical information portals, may have more rigorous inclusion criteria than other searchable websites. Examples of medical portals can be found at:

nhsdirect.nhs.uk
patient.co.uk

Links to many British medical charities will be found at the Association of Medical Research Charities (www.amrc.org.uk) and Charity Choice (www.charitychoice.co.uk).

Search phrases

Be specific when entering a search phrase. Searching for information on 'cancer' could give astrological information as well as medical: 'lung cancer' would be a better choice. Either use the engine's advanced search feature and ask for the exact phrase, or put the phrase in quotes – 'lung cancer' – as this will link the words. Adding 'uk' to your search phrase will bring up mainly British websites, so a good search would be 'lung cancer' uk (don't include uk within the quotes).

Always remember that the internet is international and unregulated. Although it holds a wealth of invaluable information, individual websites may be biased, out of date or just plain wrong. Family Doctor Publications accepts no responsibility for the content of links published in their series.

Index

ACE (angiotensin-converting enzyme) inhibitors **29**
admission to hospital **36**
anaesthetic room **38**
anaesthetics **37–8**
anaesthetist, preoperative visit **37**
anatomy of heart **3–4**
aneurysmectomy **56**
angina **11, 12, 14**
– blood tests **25**
– drug treatments **28**
– exercise tests (stress tests) **22**
– in valve disease **17**
angiography **24–5**
angioplasty (PTCA) **27, 29–31**
ankles, swollen **17**
– diuretic treatment **29**
anticoagulant therapy **59, 60, 82**
aorta **3, 4**
aortic stenosis **16**
aortic valve **7, 8**
– echocardiography **23**
– mixed disease **17**
aortic valve repair **62**
aortic valve replacement **61**
appetite after surgery **77–8**
arterial blood pressure line **38, 71, 72**
arteries **5**
– use as conduits in CABG **49–50, 50–3**
– *see also* coronary arteries
artificial heart valves **58–61**
artificial hearts **84**
ASH (Action on Smoking and Health) **86**
assessment for heart transplant **64**
atherosclerosis **11–12**
– of blood vessels to brain **44**
atria **3, 4**
– location of pacemaker **9**
atrial fibrillation **59**
– pulmonary vein ablation **68–9**
atrial septal defect (ASD) **66–7**

ball and cage valves **58, 60**
balloon angioplasty **30**
balloon pump, intra-aortic **42, 43**
balloon valvuloplasty **27, 31–2**
bathing after surgery **77**
Benefits Enquiry Line **86**
benefits of surgery **34–5**
beta blockers **28**
bi-leaflet valves **58, 60**
bleeding after surgery **43–4**
blood
– functions of **3**
– volume of **4**

blood pressure **9–10**
blood pressure monitoring **38, 72**
blood tests **25**
– before surgery **37**
blood-thinning therapy **59, 60, 82**
breastbone
– cutting for surgery **53**
– repairing after surgery **55**
– wound infections **45**
breathing difficulties
– after surgery **44–5**
– risk of wound infections **45**
breathing tube **71, 72**
breathlessness in valve disease **17**
– diuretic treatment **29**
British Heart Foundation **86**
bruising **77**

calcium antagonists **28**
cancellation of surgery **35**
capillaries **5, 6**
cardiac catheterisation (angiography) **24–5**
cardiac enzymes **25**
cardiac hypertrophy, in valve disease **16**
cardiac output (CO) **8–9**
cardiac surgeons **18**
– preoperative visit **37**
cardiologists **18**
cardioplegia **41**
cardiopulmonary bypass **38–42**
– during CABG **47, 54, 55**
– problems coming off machine **42–3**
Cath Lab **24–5**
catheters, urinary **38, 71, 72**
central lines **38, 71, 72**
cephalic vein **49**
chambers of heart **3–4**
chest
– examination of **19–20**
– how it is opened during surgery **53**
chest drains **44, 71, 72**
Chest, Heart and Stroke **86–7**
chest infections, as complication of surgery **34, 37, 45**
chest physiotherapy **75**
chest X-rays **20–1, 37**
children, heart surgery **66–7**
cholesterol tests **25**
chordae tendinae **8**
circulatory system **4–6**
circumflex coronary artery **6**
clicking, from mechanical valves **59**
clinic appointments after surgery **81–2**
clothing, what to bring into hospital **36**
colds **37**
collapse of lungs **45**
complications of surgery **33–4, 42–5**
conduits in CABG **47, 49–53**
– sewing into place **54**
confusion after surgery **44**
congenital heart disease **66–7**
consent forms
– for angioplasty **30**
– for surgery **33, 37**
constipation, after surgery **34, 78**
cooling of body during surgery **40**
coronary arteries **6**
– in ischaemic heart disease **11–14**
coronary artery bypass grafting (CABG) **47–9**
– conduits **49–53**
– follow-up after surgery **81**
– how long grafts last **55**
– how the operation is done **53–6**
– off-pump (OPCAB) **42, 47–8, 83**
– 're-do' surgery **55–6**
– support stockings **76–7**
– urgent after angioplasty **30**
cusps of heart valves **7**
cycling **80**

Dacron grafts **53**
death, risk of **34**
deep venous thrombosis (DVT) **76**
defibrillators **27, 32, 41**
deoxygenated blood **3, 4**
depression after surgery **78**
diabetes
– preparation for surgery **37**
– risk of wound infections **45**

diagnosis of heart disease **18–19**
– angiography **24–5**
– blood tests **25**
– chest X-rays **20–1**
– ECG **21–2**
– echocardiography **23–4**
– examination **19–20**
– exercise tests **22**
– history **19**
– scans **25–6**
diastolic pressure **9**
diet after surgery **78**
digoxin **29**
discharge from hospital **78–9**
discharge from wounds **77, 80**
diuretics (water tablets) **29**
dobutamine echocardiography **26**
donor organs, shortage of **64**
drains in chest cavity **44, 71, 72**
drinking
– after surgery **76, 77–8**
– avoidance before surgery **37**
drips **38, 71, 72**
driving after surgery **80–1**
drug-eluting stents **31**
drug treatments **18, 27, 28–9**
DVLA, informing them about surgery **81**
dye test (angiography) **24–5**

eating
– after surgery **77–8**
– avoidance before surgery **37**
ECG (electrocardiography) **21–2, 37**
– monitor **38, 71, 72**
echocardiography **23–4, 26**
electrophysiology **32**
emergency cases **35**
end-stage heart failure **64**
established atrial fibrillation **68**
examination by doctor **19–20**
exercise
– after leaving hospital **79–80**
– effect on heart rate **9**
– and ischaemic heart disease **12**
exercise tests **22**
exercises
– for legs and feet **77**
– for shoulders and arms **76, 80**
extubation **70, 71, 75**

family, visiting you in hospital **75**
family history **19, 25**
'fast tracking' after surgery **1, 70**
fibrillation, intermittent **41**
flu **37**
follow-up after surgery **81–2**
free grafts **53**
'furring' of arteries **11**

gas exchange **5**
gastroepiploic artery **49, 52–3**
general anaesthetic (GA) **37–8**
genetic engineering **84**
GP, as source of help after discharge **78–9, 80**
GTN (glyceryl trinitrate) **28**

headache, after GTN **28**
heart
– anatomy **3–4**
– function **8–10**
– protection during surgery **41–2, 49**
– stopping it during surgery **41**
– X-ray appearance **20**
heart attacks **11, 14**
– blood tests **25**
– effect on heart rate **9**
heart failure
– drug treatments **29**
– end-stage **64**
– in ischaemic heart disease **14**
– in valve disease **16, 17**
heart–lung machine (cardiopulmonary bypass) **38–42**
– problems coming off it **42–3**
– use during CABG **47**
heart rate (HR) **8–9**
heart transplantation **64–5**
Heart UK **87**
heart valves *see* valves
hearts, artificial **84**
help, where to find it
– searching the internet **88–9**
– useful addresses **86–8**
high-dependency unit (HDU) **74**

history **19**
'hole in the heart' **66–7**
home, return after surgery **74, 79**
hospital
– discharge from **78–9**
– length of stay **1, 74**
hospital admission, what to bring with you **36**
hygiene after surgery **77**
hypertrophy of heart in valve disease **16**

ICU (intensive care unit) **35, 70–4**
– stay after heart transplantation **65**
ICU nurse, preoperative visit **37**
immunosuppressants **65**
incompetent (leaky) valves **15–16**
intermittent fibrillation **41**
internal mammary arteries (IMAs) **49, 51**
intra-aortic balloon pump **42, 43**
intravenous pain relief **76**
ischaemic heart disease (IHD) **11–14**
– angioplasty and stenting **29–31**
– diagnosis **19, 20, 24–5**
– drug treatments **28–9**
– surgery **47–56**
ISDN (isosorbide dinitrate) **28**
ISMN (isosorbide mononitrate) **28**

keyhole surgery **69, 83**
kidney disease, risks of surgery **34**
kidney failure, as complication of surgery **34, 44**
kidney machines **73**

laser surgery to heart **56**
leaky valves **15–16**
left coronary arteries **6, 13**
left internal mammary artery (LIMA) **51**
left-sided heart failure **17**
legs, swollen **17**
– diuretic treatment **29**
loupes (magnifying spectacles) **54**
lung disease, risks of surgery **34**
lungs
– collapse of **45**
– gas exchange **5**

magnifying spectacles (loupes) **54**
mechanical heart valves **58, 59, 60**
medication after surgery **79**
minimally invasive surgery **69, 83**
mitral stenosis **16**
– balloon valvuloplasty **32**
mitral valve **7, 8**
– echocardiography **23**
mitral valve surgery **61–2**
– damage to heart conduction system **68**
mixed aortic valve disease **17**
mobilisation after surgery **76**
MRI (magnetic resonance imaging) **26**
MUGA (multi-gated acquisition) scans **25–6**
myocardial infarction *see* heart attacks
myocardial protection **41–2, 49**
myocardium **4**

National Institute for Health and Clinical Excellence (NICE) **87**
nausea after surgery **76, 77**
neck, drip in (central line) **38, 71, 72**
NHS Smoking Helpline **87**
nitrate therapy **28**
nodal ablation **32**
nuclear medicine department, scans **25–6**
numbness around wounds **80**

off-pump coronary bypass (OPCAB) **42, 47–8, 83**
operating department practitioners (ODPs) **38**
operations, duration of **1**
overweight people, risk of wound infections **45**
oxygen masks **75**
oxygen starvation of heart muscle **12**
oxygenated blood **3, 4**

pacemaker of heart **9**
pacemaker insertion **27, 32, 68**
pacing wires, temporary **62, 78**
pain relief **76**
painful wounds **80**
paralysis after stroke **44**
paralysis during surgery **38**
paroxysmal atrial fibrillation **68–9**
percussion of chest **19**
perfusionist **40, 54, 55**
pericardium **4**
– use for artificial heart valves **58**
PET (positron emission tomography) **25–6**
physical examination **19–20**
– before surgery **36**
physiotherapy **75, 79, 80**
pigs
– as source of heart valves **58, 59–61**
– xenotransplantation **84**
plaques **11, 12**
polymer heart valves **84–5**
portals **89**
positive exercise (stress) test **22**
potassium, use to stop heart **41**
pre-admission clinics **36**
premedication (pre-med) **36**
preparing for surgery **35–7**
press-ups **80**
prognostic benefits of surgery **34–5**
proximal ischaemic heart disease **14**
PTCA (percutaneous transcoronary angioplasty) **27, 29–31**
pulmonary artery and veins **3, 4**
pulmonary artery catheters **73**
pulmonary valve **7, 8**
pulmonary valve surgery **62**
pulmonary vein ablation **68–9**
pulmonary vein isolation **32**

radial artery **49, 52, 53**
radioactive markers **26**
're-do' CABG surgery **55–6**
recovery **1–2, 70, 75–6**
– depression **78**
– discharge from hospital **78–9**
– eating and drinking **77–8**
– going home **79**
– in ICU **70–4, 76**
– slow **44**
– ward stay **74, 76**
– washing **77**
redness of wounds **80**
regurgitation (leaking) of valves **15–16**
rehabilitation **74, 75–6**
– avoidance of smoking **81**
– driving **80–1**
– exercise **79–80**
– resuming sexual activity **81**
– returning to work **81**
– sleeping **80**
– *see also* recovery
relatives, visiting you in hospital **75**
rheumatic fever **17, 19**
rhythm disturbances, treatment **27, 32, 68–9**
right coronary artery **6, 13**
right internal mammary artery (RIMA) **51**
right-sided heart failure **17**
risks of surgery **33–4**
robotic assisted surgery **84**

saphenous veins **49, 50**
scans **25–6**
septum of heart **4**
– atrial septal defect **66–7**
– rupture in heart attack **56**
sexual activity, resuming after surgery **81**
shaving before surgery **36**
showering after surgery **77**
sickness after surgery **76, 77**
sleeping after surgery **80**
slow heart beat, pacemaker insertion **68**
smokers, physiotherapy **75**
smoking **34, 45**
– ASH (Action on Smoking and Health) **86**
– avoidance after surgery **81**
– NHS Smoking Helpline **87**
Smoking Quitlines (Quit) **87**
sphygmomanometer **9**
sponge treatment for wound infections **45**

starving before surgery **37**
statins **50**
stenosis
– of coronary arteries **11**
– of valves **15, 16**
stenting **27, 30–1**
steroid therapy, risk of wound infections **45**
stiffness after surgery **76**
stitches, removal of **78**
stopping the heart **41**
stress tests **22, 26**
stroke, as complication of surgery **34, 44**
Stroke Association **87–8**
stroke volume (SV) **8–9**
support stockings **76–7**
surgeon, preoperative visit **37**
surgery
– avoidance of **27**
– cancellation **35**
– in children **66–7**
– heart transplantation **64–5**
– for ischaemic heart disease **47–56**
– possible complications **33–4, 42–5**
– preparing for it **35–7**
– risks and benefits **33–5**
– for valvular heart disease **58–62**
– waiting times **35**
swallowing, painful **76**
swimming **80**
swollen ankles and legs **17**
– diuretic treatment **29**
symptomatic benefits of surgery **34**
symptoms, of ischaemic heart disease **12–14**
synthetic grafts **49, 53**
systolic pressure **9**

Teflon grafts **53**
temperature of body during surgery **40–1**
tests, before discharge from hospital **78**
thallium scans **25–6**
theatre nurses **38**
thrombosis
– in arteries **11, 12**
– in leg veins **76**
tilting disc valves **58, 60**
tiredness after surgery **75, 76**
tissue valves **58, 59–61**
total arterial revascularisation (TAR) **52**
total artificial heart (TAH) **84**
transmyocardial revascularisation (TMR) **56**
transoesophageal echocardiography (TOE) **24**
transplant surgery **64–5**
– artificial hearts **84**
– xenotransplantation **84**
transthoracic echocardiography (TTE) **23–4**
treadmill tests **22**
tricuspid valve **7, 8**
tricuspid valve surgery **62**
triple bypass operations **47**
– choice of conduits **51**
triple therapy for ischaemic heart disease **28**

ultrasound
– echocardiography **23–4**
– of neck **44**
urinary catheters **38, 71, 72**
urine, measurement of **72**

valve repair **62**
valves, artificial **58–61, 84–5**
valves of heart **6–8**
valvular heart disease **15–17**
– diagnosis **19, 20, 23**
– drug treatments **29**
– follow-up after surgery **81–2**
– surgery **58–62**
valvuloplasty **27, 31–2**
veins **5, 6**
– use as conduits in CAGB **49–50**
vena cavae **3, 4**
ventilators **38**
– going back on them after surgery **45**
– weaning off **70–1**
ventricles **3, 4**

ventricular assist devices (VADs) **42, 42–3, 84**
ventricular septal defect (VSD) repair **56**
visitors **75**

waiting times for surgery **35**
walking after surgery **79**
ward stay after surgery **74**
warfarin therapy, after valve replacement **59, 60, 82**
'warm heart surgery' **40–1**
washing after surgery **77**
water tablets (diuretics) **29**
work, return after surgery **81**
wound infections **34, 45**
– risk from synthetic grafts **53**
wounds, problems with **77, 80**

X-rays of chest **20–1, 37**
xenografts **59–61**
xenotransplantation **84**